Family Table

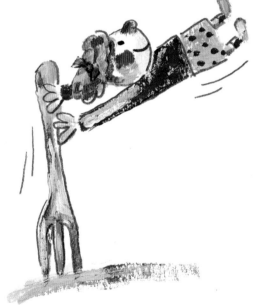

Fitzhenry and Whiteside Limited
195 Allstate Parkway
Markham, Ontario L3R 4T8

In the United States :
311 Washington Street,
Brighton, Massachusetts 02135

www.fitzhenry.ca godwit@fitzhenry.ca

Fitzhenry & Whiteside acknowledges with thanks the Canada Council for the Arts, and the Ontario Arts Council for their support of our publishing program. We acknowledge the financial support of the Government of Canada through the Book Publishing Industry Development Program (BPIDP) for our publishing activities.

Library and Archives Canada Cataloguing in Publication
Breton, Marie, 1962-
        The family table : recipes and strategies for the challenge / Marie Breton & Isabelle Emond ;
photos by Louis Prud'homme ; illustrations by Philippe Beha. Translation o : À table en famille. Includes index.
ISBN 978-1-55455-037-1
        1. Cookery. 2. Diet. I. Emond, Isabelle II. Title.
TX714.B7313 2007   641.5   C2007-904389-5

United States Cataloguing-in-Publication Data

Breton, Marie.
    The family table : recipes and strategies for the challenge / Marie Breton & Isabelle Emond ; photos by Louis Prud'homme ; illustrations by Philippe Beha.
Originally published : Quebec, QC, Canada : Flammarion, as À table en famille, 2006.
[192] p. : ill., photos. ;   cm.
Includes index.
ISBN-13 : 978-1-55455-037-1 (pbk.)
1. Cookery. 2. Diet. I. Emond, Isabelle. II. Prud'homme, Louis. III. Beha, Philippe. IV. Title.
641.5 dc22   TX714.B748 2007

Culinary stylist : Stéphan Boucher
Accessory stylist : Irène Garavelli
Studio assistant : Caroline Graf
Digital assistants : Annie Fafard and Gilles Gagné
Accessories courtesy Caban, Les Touilleurs, Quincaillerie Dante and Zone

Louis Prud'homme thanks Ulysse Arsenault-Maynard, Irène Garavelli and Thomas Prud'homme for posing for photographs.

Book Design by Olivier Lasser

Printed and bound in Singapore

1 3 5 7 9 10 8 6 4 2

MARIE BRETON AND **ISABELLE EMOND**
DIETICIANS

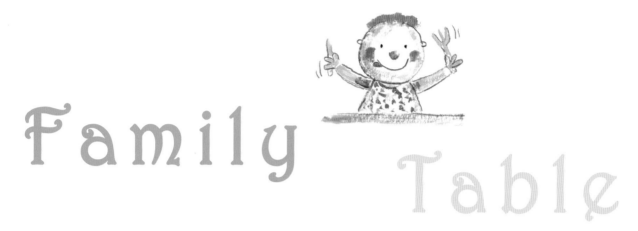

Family Table

RECIPES AND STRATEGIES

PHOTOS BY LOUIS PRUD'HOMME · ILLUSTRATIONS BY PHILIPPE BEHA

Fitzhenry & Whiteside

Contents

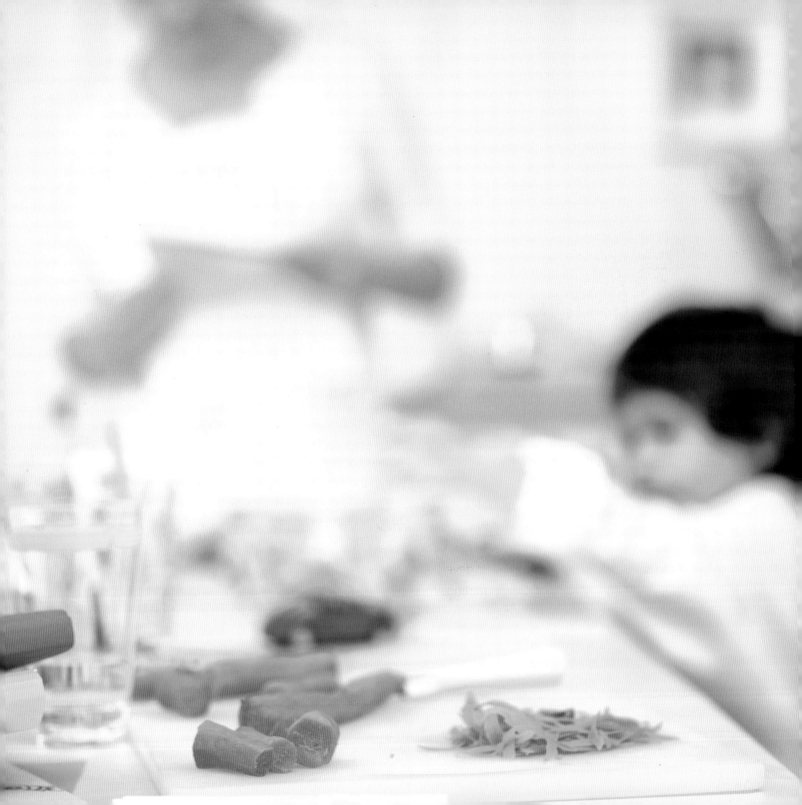

Dinner as a family is a real challenge!

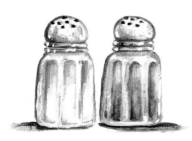

Preparing meals and sitting down to enjoy them is not so easy these days. We all work long hours. On returning home after stopping at daycare and the convenience store, we try to become parents again; to cook, supervise homework and baths, while juggling our sons' hockey practice, our daughters' singing lessons and the never-ending household chores. To top it all, our daughter hardly touches her food and sonny snubs whatever is offered. Indeed, if assembling the family around a meal is a challenge in itself, to ensure that they eat well (or simply eat at all) becomes an accomplishment! However, it is doable, and this cookbook demonstrates it.

Meals are essential to the nutritional and emotional well-being of the family. They offer the unique opportunity to re-establish contact, to exchange the day's happenings and reinforce bonds. For families who choose to make their traditional dinner a daily ritual it should not be surprising that they profit from an increased sense of family belonging. Moreover, the children of these families have a far more nutritional base than those who snack all day long or eat by themselves in front of the television. They feed themselves better at home, make wiser choices while outside the home, and develop their own tastes for a wider variety of foods. It is disquieting when our youth have such difficulties finding good nourishing food in school cafeterias and food outlets. Unfortunately, only one-third of teenagers have, at best, two weekly family meals![1]

1. D. Neumark-Sztainer, P.J. Hannan, M. Story, J. Croll and C. Perry. "Family meal patterns : associations with socio-demographic characteristics and improved dietary intake among adolescents," *J Am Diet Assoc* 103(3) : 317-22, 2003.

With no family meal, a house is only a place to live! But in spite of the evidence, many of us claim to have no time to shop, cook or sit at the table at mealtime. There are solutions, like those we offer in the following chapters. However, strategies and tools are not enough. A positive attitude is needed. A desirable attitude will allow us to find the time and make the tasks more pleasurable. To eat is necessary — but this need will be better fulfilled if one chooses to make it a priority for oneself and one's family. It is only then that you can fully benefit from the resources available.

If feeding your family well is a priority, this cookbook is for you. It supplies realistic and usable ideas to plan your menus and purchases, make healthy food choices and prepare meals efficiently. It will guide you with suggestions to help your children broaden their food selections, to consume according to their body requirements and to behave appropriately at the table. For daily inspiration, you will find approximately one hundred recipes adapted to today's realities: nourishing dishes, fast to make and good to eat (so our little tasters tell us) with no more than a dozen ingredients that are easy to find. You will also find tips, variations and nutritional input, which will make your life easier. Many of these dishes can be doubled, frozen, or prepared in part, or completely in advance. In addition, your child will be able to lend a hand, thanks to accompanying children's task suggestions.

There is no good or bad method. There are only approaches that work best according to each family. We hope you find what's best for yours.

Parents and children, it's time to gather around the table!

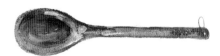

1. Developing a Good Eater

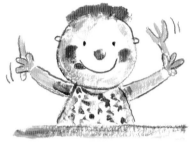

The kind of food one eats is important but the way it is presented is just as important. To encourage our children to expand their food choices, let's learn to "negotiate" with them.

A good eater is not a child who arrives famished at the table, quickly eats the plate clean and leaves overstuffed. It is not a child who eats everything (or almost) with obvious pleasure and great table manners! Does anyone like everything? A good eater eats when hungry and stops when full (even though half the chocolate cake is left). The child finds what is needed from the food offered at the table, accepts most of the food and politely turns down what is liked least. A good eater uses cutlery in an appropriate fashion, behaves agreeably and has good table manners. Of course, Rome was not built in a day. To develop such habits takes years and it forces us sometimes to review and revise our methods.

HOW TO ACT?

To raise a good eater requires a sharing of responsibilities between the parent and the child. This means each has his or her own tasks. This also implies that once work is done, one must resist the temptation to step on the other's "territory"…One must trust one's child and assume that the child will do the right thing. And it will be done.

The principle of division of responsibilities was conceived by the American dietician and psychologist Ellyn Satter more than thirty years ago. This principle is well proven and is applied by an increasing number of nutritionists the world over. The rule is simple and effective. It can be applied to all children whether sick or healthy and of all ages (with minor adjustments), according to this principle :

The parent is responsible for the what, when and where. By this we mean what food is prepared, the hour it is served and the place where it is served.

**The child is responsible for how much.
By this we mean the amount of food the child will eat from what is offered.**

The shopping is done. Nourishing meals are prepared. The table is set on time. The family gathers in an amicable atmosphere. This is our work as parents. The rest is your child's responsibility. Your child will choose what to eat (or not to eat), and how much, from the selection offered.

The word here is: trust. It is preferable to trust your child rather than to control. Learn to relax and let the process evolve. We convey trust in our children when we accept that they are no longer hungry (or are hungry) and when we accept that they decline a particular food. We question their self-knowledge when we attempt to force them to eat certain foods in certain quantities.

If we accept the principle of shared responsibility our children will develop into good eaters as they mature. They will feel understood, respected and loved when our trust is given. Many pleasant hours will be spent at the table and you will have the satisfaction of a job well done. If we perceive differently, the child will feel controlled and consequently will misbehave. The child will not feel good about him or herself, or about you. Eating habits will suffer and deteriorate. This will be the beginning or continuation of bad eating habits.

WHY?

You can lead the horse to water but you can't make it drink. We can bring the child (and the food) to the table but if we try forcing the child to eat what isn't wanted we run the risk of losing the battle. All children want to eat. They know instinctively how much their body requires for growth as per their genetic programing. Our children expect and love limits from us as parents. This creates a nurturing and positive environment, enabling them to develop physically and psychologically.

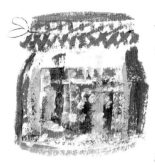

The child wants to eat. The will to live and the desire to eat are instinctive even with the sickest of children. However, some parents seem convinced that their little treasure will not survive if they don't take the upper hand. So they plead, argue, talk, force, reward, threaten, or use all sorts of blackmail to have the child swallow the smallest spoonful. On the other hand, some parents are convinced their little one is obsessed with food and if they let the child eat as much as he wants, it will lead to overindulgence and obesity. They then try to restrain the child from overeating.

The child knows what amount to eat. By paying attention to internal signals which indicate hunger or fullness, the child can adjust food intake to bodily demands, and there is no need to intervene. Her body knows what amount is appropriate. This was also the way for us before we were subjected to all sorts of doctrines and myths which kept changing from time to time according to the style and edict of the day.

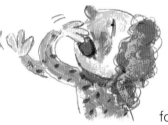

The child naturally resists anything new. Children are cautious when faced with unknown foods. They do not like whatever is new so rarely accept it the first time around. Neophobia is at its maximum until a child is three years old and only time and repeat exposure will win him over. So what is important is not that Johnny eats broccoli tonight but that he eats it some day and for the rest of his life. He has within himself the motivation to experiment with new foods. He sees his parents eat different foods. There is no need for additional pressure.

The child needs time. Waiting is what is hardest for parents. We must stop speaking or acting when we see our child (once again) choose the same foods, hardly touching the plate or only eating the bread. This is how we will give the child the chance to select a broader variety of food.

Children react badly to pressure. Almost all parents persist in pressuring because they want immediate results. They are often doing what their parents did before them. This pressure comes from good intentions.

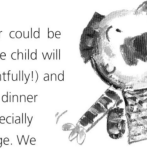

- **What if we force the child to eat?** If we do anything that resembles or could be perceived by the child as an obligation to eat, the child senses this. Generally the child will resist. If the parent further insists, the child rebels and doesn't eat (or eats resentfully!) and the vicious cycle continues. The result: the parent feels guilty, the child sulks, the dinner table becomes a combat zone and the situation deteriorates. Some children (especially the very young) enjoy refusing food and later use this game to their own advantage. We can encourage a child to taste new foods but should never force it.

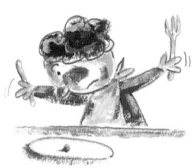

- **What if we restrict the child's eating?** If we try to restrict a child from eating (to keep her thin for example), the child feels that food is being denied and becomes preoccupied with it. If the opportunity presents itself, the child will challenge you or will eat out of fear of being hungry. At the same time, a child who is regularly denied food which is considered "desirable," will demand it even more. As soon as the opportunity arises she will overindulge out of the fear of missing out!

- **One way or the other,** by being continually forced or denied, the child loses his instinct to detect the internal signals of hunger, appetite and satiety. The child will not consume the desirable amount of food and perhaps will not grow according to the norm. The child also does not learn to appreciate good food and is tempted by less healthy choices ...

Children do not need rewards. They are not stupid. They know when they are being manipulated or pressured, even if it is done with subtlety. The American psychologist Leann Birch, in one of her studies, gave a reward to a group of children for having tried a new food. In the control group, on the other hand, she let the children choose and gave no reward. It is interesting to learn that the children given the reward were later less likely than the second group to try that food again. Other studies have demonstrated that when we use a certain food as a reward for eating another food, in the eyes of the child the value of the reward food is enhanced and the desire for it increases. If we reward Jane with dessert for having eaten broccoli, we have taught her to like dessert more and broccoli less.[2]

2. L.L. Birch, D.W. Marlin and J. Rotter. "Eating as the "means" activity in a contingency: Effects on young children's food preference", *Child Development,* 55(2) : 431-9, 1984.

A DAILY ROUTINE

Here, in greater detail, is how to apply the principle of the division of responsibilities. These proven techniques will allow you to avoid the usual traps and will prevent potential conflicts around the table. In short:

bring meals to the table,
take pleasure in having meals as a family,
let the children do the rest.

Choosing the menu. We are the food guardians. It is up to us to decide what food comes into the house (or not) and what will be served at the table. After all, we know best about food and what our children need for growth. It is the child's responsibility to adjust to the family rituals and not for the family to bend to the child's tastes and demands. Consequently, all members of the family should be offered the same thing, but no one is obligated to eat all that is presented!

It is not essential that all foods brought to the table please everyone at the same time. Unfortunately in many families the selection ends up being limited by the demands of family members. This said, it makes sense to plan meals which will combine loved, familiar foods (which include the child's favorite dishes from time to time) with foods the child is less familiar with. If, for example, we have planned a meal with a meat that is not very popular, we can include a preferred vegetable and also a food (such as bread) on which the child will be able to satisfy her hunger. By offering several dishes to choose from, we respect the child's tastes and strong dislikes without having to prepare something else to please her.

If our little ones do not accept automatically all that is offered, they will in time, because these foods will often be on the table and they will see that several members of the family enjoy them. In fact, children often end up adopting our eating habits and tastes. In the meantime, if your children do not want to eat their meal that is their choice. We must not feel guilty or responsible. Let's remember: our work is over when the food arrives on the table, not in the child's tummy…

Do not offer another choice. It would be so easy to bring butter, peanut butter or the child's preferred cereal when he is not interested in what has been prepared. But, in doing so, no one benefits. The child who is offered an easy solution is encouraged in his attitude. If he does not learn to eat his meals he is sent the message that he does not have to. Rather than taking a risk on something new or eating like the rest of the family, he returns to a sure thing: what he knows and cherishes.

The family meal gives us the opportunity to introduce new foods. When parents submit to the child's whims, the child continues to restrict her tastes and preferences. This is the opposite of what we are trying to achieve. Even the most indulgent of parents ends up one day being fed up with submitting to the demands of their offspring. They then begin to insist that the child eat what is presented but doesn't want to eat it. Johnny is not happy? He will be hungry enough to eat what is offered at the next meal. Meanwhile, with a variety of food being offered at the table, the child can select enough to sustain himself, unless he is simply not hungry.

Establish a regular schedule. To be nourished is a primary human need. It is reassuring for a child to know that meals will come at regular times; that he will have enough food and will not starve. Scheduled meals and snacks will give the child this security. Regular mealtimes also allow the child to better control his hunger and sense of being full. If a child is allowed to snack any time on what he pleases, you run the risk that the child will have no appetite when a nourishing meal is presented. By following a regular schedule he will feel hungry (but not starving) by dinner time and will have a healthy interest in what is on the table. To have a regular schedule for meals and snacks, we avoid the child's desire to snack constantly.

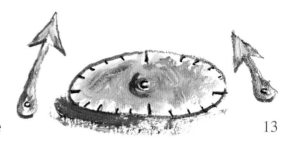

Have realistic expectations. A small child eats often with her fingers. A preschooler uses a fork and spoon…and fingers. The cup of milk may still get spilled. A teenager may still demand that you remove "uncool" food from her plate. It takes time before a child eats properly and is able to handle most foods. Be tolerant and don't get too preoccupied with the behavior. Instead, keep the paper towels handy!

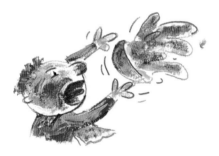

Don't hesitate to express your expectations. A child's manners do not have to be sophisticated, but acceptable enough that mealtimes run smoothly. Otherwise, the child will have to leave the table. Let the child know that criticisms, complaints and poor manners are not acceptable. Balancing on the chair, throwing food or making unappetizing noises is not acceptable! We say "yes," "please" and "no thank you" and sit firmly on our butts.

Here are some unacceptable behaviors:
- Whining or complaining about the food.
- Eating with mouth open or making noises.
- Slouching in the chair or leaning on the table.
- Wiping mouth (or blowing nose) with sleeve or tablecloth.
- Licking knife or plate.
- Being impolite.
- Throwing food.
- Balancing on the chair.
- Speaking with a mouthful of food.
- Eating standing or half seated.

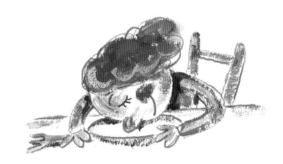

Set an example. Our children want to eat and they want to eat the same things we do. But they need time and our perseverance along the way. We can help by offering opportunities to try new flavors and by acting the way we would expect them to behave one day. Our children observe what we eat and are influenced by what they see. If we eat peas, eating peas eventually becomes the acceptable thing for them to do. So let's take pleasure in eating our peas. However, let us not expect our children to immediately accept whatever is set in front of them.

Persevere. Most kids love candies, fries and pop right away! But to love vegetables takes time…chances are slim that Johnny will eat artichokes in vinaigrette the first time he sees you eat them. Not even the second time. But the idea is planted. After seeing artichokes on his plate and seeing us enjoying them, he will get the idea that it must be good, that it is normal to eat them and that one day he will too. At the beginning you will feel you have gone to all this work for nothing. He may not want to even see "the thing" near his plate. Then one day he will allow you to serve him "the thing" but will not touch it. Another day, he will take a mouthful but will spit it out. Later yet he will take a mouthful but will not have any more. Then one day — Hallelujah! He will like it! Research has shown that a child may try a new food 10, 15 or 20 times in as many meals before he appreciates it. The more he is exposed to the food, the more familiar the food becomes, and the more he learns to like it.

Stay neutral. Blackmail, threats and begging have no place at the table. They ruin mealtime atmosphere and poison relationships with children. This behavior only promotes the very opposite of what you are trying to achieve. A child behaves better feeling in control. Don't attempt to force the child to eat. However, don't restrict the child from doing so. Simply bring the food to the table and let her eat according to her likes and appetite. You will find that healthy foods become more tempting when one is not forced to eat them, and nothing is more desirable than when it is forbidden. One tip: mention to your little ones that the asparagus or mussels are "grown up food" and see their interest grow at once.

Eat as a family. It is not easy to be at the table together. There are many obstacles — working days are long. School and professional extracurricular activities are often scheduled at the end of the day. But to feed your family well, meals around the table are essential. This ensures that your children have the needed essential nutrients for growth, both at home and outside, and enables them to acquire a taste for a greater variety of foods.

Mealtime is one of those rare occasions in the day when the whole family can be together again. By insisting that we all sit at the table tells our children that this together time is expected and that the family is important to us. This is not the time to watch television or settle our internal issues…ideally, it is when the children are young that we must initiate the ritual of family meals so when they are teenagers they will arrange their daily sport and school activities without forgetting the family tradition of meals.

Make mealtime pleasant. Children, like adults, need a relaxed atmosphere while they are eating. When the atmosphere at mealtime is negative, children may be reluctant to experiment with new foods, and may lose a sense of hunger and appetite. Stress can cause children to eat too much or not enough. Let's turn off the television, encourage a stimulating and engaging conversation, help children to help themselves, respect their independent choices and listen to them when they say they are no longer hungry. In short, let's focus on the pleasures of eating and being together rather than on our children's plate.

Look for variety. Even if your child has not developed a wide range of food choices it is important to emphasize variety when preparing the meal!

- **For health reasons.** Our understanding of the link between nutrition and health is far from complete and is evolving constantly. Produce a variety of menus rather than following the latest trends, thus reducing the risk of poor nutrition.

- **For pleasure.** Studies have shown that children grow tired of even their favorite foods. Why? Because taste is important to them. They eat because they enjoy it, not because they have to. Unfortunately adults are not as in tune with their internal signals. When they think they should eat a certain food they eat it whether it is good or bad. As adults, why don't we cultivate an attitude of curiosity regarding food, like our kids, just for the pleasure?

- **To develop taste.** How can we like what we do not know! For children to appreciate a variety of foods, they first have to be exposed to an assortment of foods. Conversely, if they are always served the same thing, their taste will be naturally limited…to what they know. Your child loves apples? Give her apples, but also try kiwis, mandarins, peaches, pears and tutti frutti!

Do not forbid dessert. "No veggies, no dessert," "Finish your plate first," "Five spoonfuls left"…Generations of well-intentioned parents have harassed their children with these words. Generations of children have eaten their meat and veggies by obligation and their dessert as a reward. Children's aversion to healthy food develops at the same time as their liking for sweets, to have the "right" to their dessert some children will go as far as eating twice as much as they want – the first by cleaning their plate when they are no longer hungry, the second when they eat their dessert! This was the case of a little girl who, when she was full after her main course, forced herself to throw up so she could claim her "reward." Whether a child chooses to eat or not to eat the meal the child should always be entitled to dessert, in a reasonable portion. The child will still be hungry, but next time will think twice before pushing back her plate.

Do not forbid sweets. Forbidden foods lose their attraction when they become available. From time to time, include ice cream, crackers and biscuits on the menu if they are favorites and let the child enjoy them. They will stop eating when they are no longer hungry. The children will then relax because they know these treats will be available again in future. Furthermore, if children are given quality nutrition on a regular basis, to have the occasional break from this is not necessarily bad. When choosing sweets pick those that are regular rather than those reduced in fat, sugar, calories and taste…as they satisfy the appetite and less will be consumed.

Serve tasty meals. Young children do not necessarily eat what they should eat as most adults do. They eat because it tastes good! To be a success, a meal must satisfy a child's hunger and appetite. If he does not appease his hunger, the child will not be satisfied and he will tend to later look for a snack to replace what he didn't eat at mealtime. If we want our children to enjoy food, we will have to cook more often. And let's face it – commercial products cannot compete, taste-wise, with homemade food.

Restaurant meals

If you rarely go to a restaurant, you can afford to ignore nutritional choices and let your child eat what she wishes. On the other hand, if you go often you will have to give some guidelines to help her make wise choices. You could, for example, ask the child to have at least three of the food groups* in her meal (fries and ketchup do not count as vegetables!): a hamburger with a glass of milk, a pizza or chicken nuggets with a salad and juice for example. Another possibility is to allow her only one indulgence: pop, fries, turnover, milkshake or other food of her choice.

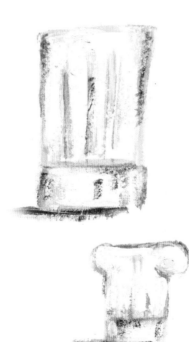

* The four food groups: cereal and grains, fruits and vegetables, dairy products, and meats and alternatives.

18

Phrases to avoid:

"Eat because it's good for you."

"Make mommy happy and eat."

"Five more spoonfuls and you can leave the table."

"Okay, but you won't have any dessert."

"If you eat, you can have a candy."

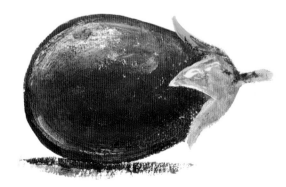

2. Get organized

I n this chapter we will learn how to get organized. Organize work and storage spaces, menus, inventories, shopping lists and trips to the grocery store…a full but promising program !

It is not easy to plan meals and shopping lists, do the shopping, and then cook and clean up, especially with children about. This takes discipline, determination and a strong conviction that it is best for your family. The suggestions made here will lighten your task and will transform hard labor into a satisfying activity.

WORK SPACE

There is a risk that children in the kitchen might burn or cut themselves. You could of course, keep the little ones out of the kitchen, but we believe it is preferable to make the kitchen a safer and more functional place and keep the kids involved.

Avoid danger. Keep sharp knives out of the reach of children; store knives in a butcher block for instance. Never leave them lying about on the counter! On the stovetop use the back elements first and turn pan handles toward the back so that swift little hands cannot reach them.

Plan work islands. Here are some ideas:
- **A preparation corner:** here you can gather measuring cups, cooking utensils, mixing bowls, and basic dry goods (flour, sugar, brown sugar). Place dry ingredients in closed containers where they will be easier to measure than from their original bags. The most often used utensils (ladle, spatula, wooden spoon, wire whisk) can be assembled in a metal box or jar on the counter or suspended above the island or a hook on the wall. They will be easier to reach than when placed at the bottom of a drawer, especially if our hands are full of butter or flour.

- **A cooking corner:** here we gather baking sheets, cake and muffin tins and cooking dishes in the drawer below the range or, if this is full, in a cupboard nearby.

- **A fruit and vegetable corner:** this is where we store the vegetable peeler, vegetable brush, cutting board and plastic knives for kids near the sink where fruits and vegetables are washed and prepared.

- **A kid's corner:** it could be a cupboard in which childproof plastic bowls and containers can be stored. You may allow the child to wash the carrots or have fun in the sink filling and emptying glasses and cups with water. A plastic container full of raw rice with measuring cups can also work wonders. This said, no matter what we choose to let a child play with, we have to expect that his attention will not last long and we can't expect him to be of great help. We see this kind of children's participation as an investment in the future.

STORAGE SPACE

Some foods keep better at room temperature. Others keep better in the fridge or freezer, whereas other foods keep better in fresh, dry and well-ventilated spaces. In spite of the best conditions, even the so-called non-perishable foods like preserves, pasta, flour or corn syrup do not last forever. The following suggestions will help you avoid food spoilage and lost shopping dollars.

Consider the purchase of a freezer. This investment will allow you to purchase more at once and shop less often, take advantage of bargains and to cook ahead or in large quantities. The freezer compartment of your refrigerator will thank you for it.

Plan a cold room or a corner in the garage (where weather permits). These cold spaces (ideally between 7°C and 10°C [45°F and 50°F]) are perfect to keep carrots, onions, apples, and preserves for several weeks or even months, and are ideal for rapid cooling of spaghetti sauce or soup. However, the temperature will not be cold enough to leave perishable food (dairy products, meats, eggs, etc.) for more than four hours. By keeping only small quantities in the kitchen and the remainder in the cold room, we free up our kitchen space.

Use free basement or cupboard space. The newfound shelves will quickly pay for themselves thanks to the savings acquired when buying flour, sugar, pasta and rice or preserves in bulk and other less perishable foods found on sale. This space must be well ventilated, fresh and dry. It is best to avoid locations above the stove or close to a heater or furnace.

Use a thermometer in the refrigerator and in the freezer. Check the temperature of the fridge regularly so the proper temperature is maintained, which should be 4°C (39°F) or slightly less, and that of the freezer should be at least minus 18°C (0°F).

Inspect the refrigerator, freezer and pantry regularly. Once a week throw out perishable foods or leftovers which have been in the refrigerator for several days. Check the freezer every three months and the pantry once a year.

THE BAG METHOD

Marie always had trouble finding her way through the mess in her refrigerator and freezer. That was before her friend Christine suggested the bag method! It is simple. In well-labeled plastic bags, group similar foods – frozen vegetables, frozen fruits, raw meats, cooked meats, bread leftovers, etc – as if they were filed in a drawer. The result is that rather than emptying the freezer to find your peas you go directly to your frozen vegetables bags.

MEAL PLANNING

Meal planning may not be the most exciting of occupations. You have to stop, think, research and make a list. But believe me, there is something worse than meal planning and that is doing no meal planning. It is already bad enough by late afternoon to feel hurried, exhausted and hungry without wondering "what are we going to have for dinner?" Good planning allows us to better survive these peak times. We will be less irritable, especially with the children, and we will take more pleasure in cooking and eating as a family. We also increase our chances of producing a nutritional and tasty meal. You are probably thinking: "Another list of things to do!," "How do I know if I will feel like eating tacos on Tuesday?" "Will we be at home that evening?" It is true that the best of tools poorly used is of very little help. To be advantageous, meal planning must be realistic and respond to our needs.

Three methods, three styles

Here are the three proven methods for meal planning, each one responding to different needs. It is up to you to choose which one will suit your needs best.

Have handy:
- Family weekly timetable.
- Inspirational sources (recipe books, magazines, books or websites).
- Paper or copies of your personalized shopping list (see pg 28) and a pencil.

1. The cyclical menu

Managers of food services in hospitals, daycare centers, and drop-in centers understand the advantages of cyclical menus, from both a practical and an economical point of view. The length of the cycle varies from one to six weeks or more in places whose people stay for extended periods of time.

How do you do it? Plan two, three or four weeks of menus that you can keep in protective plastic covers and re-use in rotation for the season or the year. The cycle must be sufficiently long to offer a healthy variety. To simplify food shopping, note each week's menu directly on the personalized shopping list.

For whom? This is for those who have a regular schedule and who work best when all is meticulously planned.

2. The weekly menu

How to go about it? Once a week, during the weekend for instance, we sketch out the menus for the following week on a sheet of paper or directly on the personalized shopping list. It could be the main dish for the next three days or the complete day's menu if that works best for you. At the end of the week, the personalized shopping list can be saved for a week of menus in the future.

For whom? This is for those of us whose schedules fluctuate and change over time, or those of us who like more flexibility in our menus — most of us!

3. The daily menu

How to go about it? The day before (preferably) or on the same day, we plan the evening meal based on family tastes, time availability and what we have on hand. A well-stocked pantry is an asset!

For whom? This is for those who like to be guided by their inspiration, who have the time, an unpredictable schedule and for those who manage and control their stress well.

Is our menu completed?

Don't forget to note the name of the book and the page where the selected recipes come from. If they are on separate sheets, keep them together so their handy.

23

Six strategies

Whether we plan meals for a day or a month, the same recommendations apply.

1. **Each meal should contain a protein, a starchy food and vegetables.** It is the ideal selection for sustaining balanced menus. For starchy foods you can choose potatoes, pasta, rice or simply bread. Vegetables could be in the form of salads, veggies, tomato juice, soup or hot vegetables (consult the section "What is a good meal?" pg 38)

2. **Favor the "all in one."** These "all in one" meals combine starchy foods (rice, pasta or potatoes), vegetables and proteins (meat, eggs or legumes) while guaranteeing a complete meal that saves time and cleanup. Several such dishes are prepared ahead of time. Some examples: Mexican Roasted Chicken and Vegetables (pg 121), Broccoli Frittata (pg 161), East Indian Chickpeas (pg 156), and Red Kidney Bean Chili (pg 125).

3. **Vary colors, flavors and textures.** Would a poached fish fillet served with white sauce, mashed potatoes and cauliflower appeal to you? Would you prefer that same fillet of fish with tomato sauce, onions and black olives (Catalan Fish, pg 136), accompanied with a green salad, steamed broccoli and peach crisp? You guessed it… to see, to taste, to smell, to touch and to hear …all have their part to play in the pleasure of eating.

4. **Always avoid serving the same thing.** There is nothing wrong with repeating successful recipes. After all, it is repetition which enhances familiarization and in turn acceptance by the children. However, even the best spaghetti or shepherd's pie loses its attraction when served once too often. For health and pleasure don't slip into the "same food different day" syndrome. To achieve this, plan at least two meals without meat and two meals with fish weekly. Look through magazines, cookbooks and on the internet for new recipes.

5. **Balance preparation times.** Does the main course require lengthy preparation time? To balance this, plan to serve frozen vegetables or a mix of prewashed greens, and for dessert, choose a can of peaches or edges of fresh fruit served on toothpicks. They will go like hot cakes!

6. **Take a break.** You can easily plan to cook three nights a week. The other two nights (when family activities are planned, for example) you can opt for "the freezer find," or "leftover night," or go out to a restaurant (see below). During the weekend make a habit of preparing two meals for the week. Cook smart by doubling the recipes and freezing for a quick meal. Finally, one night a week why not empower the children by giving them carte blanche in their menu choice?

A Holiday From Dinner

There are nights when, in spite of all your planning and best intentions, you don't like eating what is planned; you are not inclined to think about eating (or even think at all!) and have no desire to cook. Here are some survival options for such times (hopefully fleeting ones)…

Leftover night. Place cold leftovers on the table and each person can compose his or her own meals and put them in the microwave. Everyone will have a different meal but at least all will eat and it will clear up the fridge. Why not take advantage of Friday nights to empty the fridge?

Explore the freezer. Lasagna, meat pies, soups, casseroles…all can go directly from the freezer to the oven or microwave and in turn to the table. This option is only valid if they have been prepared and stored in the freezer in the first place! There are also many ready-to-serve products on the market that you can keep on hand (see chapter 4, "Choose Your Foods," pg 44).

Eat at a restaurant. There are advantages to dining out — the family is seated together (a major event) where they can relax and chat and each family member makes his or her own choice. They can select what they feel like eating and then calmly wait to be served while sipping a drink and nibbling on bread; and above all everyone enjoys a meal prepared by someone else! So pile everyone into the car and pay several times over the price of a homemade meal. Sometimes it just feels good!

Order in or pick up prepared food. This gives us a break from the dishes, preparing a meal, and more time for homework or baths or simply an occasion to do nothing.

Indulge. What if we have an irresistible desire for a grilled cheese sandwich, hot dog, peanut butter sandwich, or even cereal or toast? This will not kill us. It is better to indulge in such choices with pleasure rather than feeling frustrated by having to always prepare nutritiously perfect meals. Cereal, toast and even hot dogs have some nutritional value.

PLANNING THE GROCERY SHOPPING

To plan grocery shopping ahead of time takes a while but it is time well spent. When you don't plan, you impulse buy, you forget essential ingredients, forcing a return to the grocery store during the week or a change in the menu.

Basic Inventory

With good reserves at home, you will never be short. The following is a complete inventory. It will allow for the preparation of most recipes. It can be used as is or may inspire you to develop your own inventory. Make an inventory list to be used as a reference when shopping.

The Shopping List

Method 1

Have on hand:

- Recipes for the week.
- A copy of your personalized basic inventory or the basic inventory supplied on pgs 26-27.
- A marker.

Each week, make a copy of your basic inventory which will become your shopping list. As foods disappear from the pantry and fridge, underline the needed purchases, and the ingredients to make menus for the week, indicating the amounts necessary. Before leaving, go over the list one last time to make sure nothing has been forgotten. A fine touch would be to organize your basic inventory based on the arrangement of the grocery store aisles and to follow the aisle pattern with your cart.

26

Fresh Fruits and Vegetables

Fruits

Apples
Apricots
Bananas
Berries (strawberries, raspberries, blueberries, cranberries)
Cantaloup
Grapefruit
Grapes (red, green)
Honeydew melons
Lemons (+ juice)
Limes (+ juice)
Mandarin oranges
Nectarines
Oranges
Peaches
Pears
Pineapple
Plums

Fresh vegetables and herbs

Asparagus
Avocado
Basil
Beans
Broccoli
Cabbage (+ grated)
Carrots (baby, grated)
Cauliflower
Celery
Cucumber
Eggplant
Endive
Garlic
Ginger
Green onion

Leeks
Lemongrass
Lettuce
Mushrooms
Onion (yellow, Spanish, red)
Parsley
Peppers
Potatoes
Prepared vegetables
Radishes
Shallots
Spinach
Sprouts
Sweet potato
Tomatoes (fresh, cherry, dried)
Turnip
Winter squash
Zucchini

Bread and Quick Breads

Bagels
Baguette
Buns (hot dog, hamburger)
English muffins
Muffins
Paninis
Pitas
Pizza crust
Sliced bread
Tortillas

Meats and Fish (fresh, frozen)

Bacon
Beef (ground, roast, steak, stewing meat)
Chicken (ground, whole, breast, drumsticks, stewing meat)

Deli meats
Fish (sole, haddock, salmon, trout)
Ham
Pork (ground, roast, chops, stewing meat)
Sausage
Turkey (ground, whole, cubed)

Vegetarian Products (refrigerated)

Hummus
Prepared meals
Soup
Soy desserts
Soy sausage and other veggie deli
Tofu
Veggie pâté
Veggie pies (millet and seitan)

Miscellaneous Ingredients

Baking powder
Baking soda
Bouillon (beef, chicken, vegetable)
Chocolate pudding
Cocoa powder
Cornstarch
Crumbs (bread, graham)
Dried fruit (raisins, prunes, dates, apricots, cranberries)
Evaporated milk
Dried legumes (chickpeas, white beans, lentils)
Flour (white, whole wheat, pastry)
Honey

Mixes (muffin, pie dough)
Molasses
Nuts (walnuts, almonds, peanuts, pine nuts)
Seeds (sesame, poppy, sunflower)
Sugar (white, brown, icing)
Syrup (maple, corn)
Unflavored gelatin
Vanilla
Wine (white, red)

Cereals

Bran
Cheerios
Cornflakes
Granola
Hot cereals (rolled oats, Cream of wheat, oat bran)
Rice Crispies
Shredded Wheat

Pasta and Grains

Barley
Bulgur
Couscous
Fettuccini
Lasagna
Macaroni
Popping corn
Rice (white, brown)
Spaghetti
Tapioca

Condiments and Seasonings

Dried herbs and spices: basil, bay leaf, cardamom, cayenne, chervil, chili powder, cinnamon, citrus zest, cloves, coriander (cilantro), crushed red pepper, cumin, curry, dill, garlic powder, ginger, hot mustard powder, mint, nutmeg, onion powder and flakes, oregano, paprika, parsley, pepper, rosemary, sage, salt, tarragon, thyme, turmeric
Capers
Jam
Ketchup
Mayonnaise
Mustard (yellow, Dijon)
Oil (olive, canola, peanut)
Peanut butter
Pesto
Pickles (cornichons, beets, onions, olives)
Relish
Salad dressing
Salsa
Sauce (soy, Worcestershire, Tabasco, chili)
Vinaigrette
Vinegar (white, wine, cider, balsamic, rice)

Biscuits and Crackers

Cones
Cookies (figs, dates)
Crackers
Croutons
Graham crackers
Granola bars
Rusks
Tea Biscuits

Canned Produce

Fruits
Apple sauce
Fruit salad
Mandarin oranges
Peaches
Pears
Pineapple

Vegetables
Artichoke hearts
Carrots
Corn (kernel, creamed)
Green beans
Mixed vegetables
Mushrooms
Peas
Tomatoes (whole, diced, crushed, paste, sauce)

Fish
Anchovies
Mussels (+ smoked)
Oysters (+ smoked)
Salmon
Sardines
Shrimp
Tuna
Tuna salad

Soups
Canned stock (chicken, beef, vegetable)
Creamed soups (celery, chicken, mushroom, tomato)
Lentil
Minestrone
Pea

Legumes
Bean salad
Beans in tomato sauce
Chick peas
Chili
Green beans
Lentils

Juices and Drinks

Coffee (instant, ground)
Fruit juices (apple, orange, grape)
Herbal tea
Soy drink
Tea
Vegetable juices (tomato, carrot, vegetable)
Water (spring, sparkling)

Dairy Products and Eggs

Brick cheese
Butter or margarine
Buttermilk
Cheddar cheese (grated, slices, string)
Cottage cheese
Cream (10%, 18%, 35%, aerosol)
Cream cheese
Eggs
Feta cheese
Goat cheese
Gouda cheese
Milk (1%, 2%, 3.25%)
Mozzarella (grated, slices, string)
Parmesan cheese
Ricotta cheese
Sour cream
Yogurt

Frozen Produce

Fish
Fruit (strawberries, raspberries, blueberries, cranberries, mixed)
Ice cream
Juice from concentrate
Pancakes and crepes
Popsicles
Prepared meals
Vegetables (corn, peas, broccoli, spinach, mixed)
Waffles

Paper Products and Cleaners

Aluminum foil
Bleach
Detergents (dish, dishwasher)
Freezer bags
Garbage bags
Paper (parchment, waxed)
Paper serviettes
Paper towels
Plastic wrap
Sandwich bags

Method 2

Have on hand:

- Recipes for the week.
- A copy of your personalized shopping list below.
- A pencil.

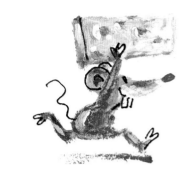

Review the ingredients needed for this week's recipes. Note in the appropriate sections what you are missing and what must be bought in necessary quantities.

PERSONALIZED SHOPPING LIST

Recipes for the week

MONDAY: _____

TUESDAY: _____

WEDNESDAY: _____

THURSDAY: _____

FRIDAY: _____

SATURDAY: _____

SUNDAY: _____

Groceries to Purchase

Fruits and vegetables	Dairy products
Cereal products	Frozen produce
Meats	Non-perishables

SHOPPING

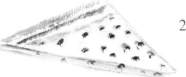

Once a month — Basic products

This is to shop for non-perishable food and kitchen items (canned goods, dry goods, cleaning supplies and paper products) for the month. You may also wish to purchase bread and milk and freeze them.

For these monthly purchases a superstore is preferable even if you have to go a little further afield. Here you can generally find name-brand merchandise in bulk at good prices. Such an expedition takes time and energy and because you will have to store all the purchases when you get home, it is best to go without the children. At home you can always ask for their help bringing the bags into the house.

By buying non-perishable foods in bulk, we not only save money but do not run the risk of running short of flour or sugar in the middle of a recipe, and we also cut down on the number of weekly visits to the grocery store.

Once a week — Perishable products

Once a week we buy milk, bread, meats, fresh fruits and vegetables as well as specific ingredients needed for the weeks recipes. Since the basic products have already been purchased, this visit is relatively short and you could take the kids along.

For more frequent weekly shopping it's best to go grocery shopping close to home, to the grocery store of your choice. With time, we know where the products are displayed. This allows us to complete our shopping as soon as possible at a lesser cost. It is proven that the longer you stay in a grocery store the more you buy! It may be tempting to run from one store to the next in search of the best buys, but when you consider the extra time and additional gas required, one wonders if there is any real benefit.

During the week — The convenience store

When necessary we can make a quick visit to the supermarket or corner convenience store to pick up milk or bread as needed.

MEAL PREPARATION

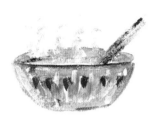

Cooking makes all the difference. Very few mass-produced meals can compete with homemade meals from a taste, nutrition and cost standpoint. Very few meals bring as much physical and emotional satisfaction as homemade meals. Unfortunately, aside from the time factor, not everybody has the same interest or the necessary skills in cooking. For some, to make soup is a real hardship and for others it is a satisfying and fulfilling activity. But can this be sustained when the task is repeated day after day? The best way to undertake meal preparation is to do it with a positive attitude and the desire to live this moment as pleasantly as possible. Here are some suggestions.

Be motivated. Cooking delicious dishes may prove a source of self-actualization, pride and the love of sharing. It can also be a relaxing hobby for one or for a couple. Devoting much of your precious time to feed your family well is a wonderful way to show that family is important. And it's a way for you to lead by example. By seeing Mom and Dad take pleasure in cooking, your child will develop his own interest in food and the skills to prepare it.

Set realistic goals. If we manage to make one more recipe per week, this will be fine. Little by little, encouraged by success, we will take on the challenge to devote more time to cooking in the evening or on the weekend.

Begin with simple recipes. There is nothing wrong with beginning with dishes that are familiar or attractive whether it be macaroni and cheese, shepherd's pie or meatloaf. After all, it does not have to be complicated to taste good!

Improve your technique. We always take more pleasure in practicing an activity in which we have some skills. Cooking is no exception. We can improve these skills by watching cooking shows on television, reading illustrated techniques in recipe books or by taking cooking courses from an accredited school. Some kitchen specialty stores, food chains and the houseware section of department stores offer cooking courses for adults and children.

Find inspiration. Leafing through magazine cooking sections, searching the internet or finding an exciting recipe book are some of the many ways to find inspiration and whet your appetite.

Manage your day. Do you take time to have breakfast, have a decent lunch and a sustaining snack in the afternoon? Do you give yourself a break? We cannot give to our family and our children if we do not take care of ourselves. By taking a break during the day, you will have more energy for the evening and you will teach your kids that you also have needs.

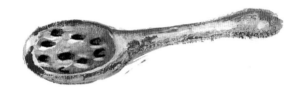

Cuisine 101

We all have our own techniques that makes us more efficient in the kitchen. Try some of ours. Perhaps you will profit by them.

Read the recipe the night before (preferably), or in the morning. Ensure that you have all the ingredients. Take out the non-perishable ingredients and cooking utensils and set them on the counter. Then remove the meats and other frozen foods from the freezer and place them in the refrigerator to thaw.

Double the recipe. Whether it is a soup, casserole, cake, muffin, or any other dish, cook it once and enjoy it twice! You freeze the extra dish for a future occasion.

Cook in two steps. If you don't have time to complete a recipe in its entirety, cut the needed ingredients, measure, mix them if applicable, cover and refrigerate. At meal time proceed with the actual cooking.

Cook in good company. It is not only efficient (you share the job and recipe preparations) but this also provides good companionship and sharing of good times with a colleague, friend, or family member.

Stock up on hamburger meat. It is an absolute necessity for meat sauces, spaghetti sauce, chilies, casseroles, soups, meat loaves and meatballs, etc. Divide the quantity bought in half-kilogram portions, put them in freezer bags, flatten and freeze them. The meat will then take less space in the freezer and will defrost faster.

Precook meatballs. Cook the meatballs (to shape them, use an ice cream scoop) on a baking sheet in a 180°C (350°F) preheated oven. Spread them out on waxed paper, on the baking sheet, allowing individual freezing, and when frozen pack them in freezer bags.

32 **Precut the meat.** Buy several kilos of meat or poultry on sale, cut them into strips or cubes according to the dish to be prepared and freeze the quantity required in labeled freezer bags. All you need to do is defrost them prior to putting them directly into the pan.

Marinate chicken breasts ahead. Spread them on a tray to freeze them separately, and transfer them into freezer bags.

Choose turkey over chicken. Cook it once and you have enough for several meals (soups, sandwiches, salads, pâtés, casseroles, fried rice, frittatas, etc.). Freeze the cooked poultry in freezer bags in portions large enough for a meal or a recipe.

Cook a large quantity of rice. Divide it and put it in plastic containers and freeze. When ready for use, defrost in the microwave oven (by adding first one or two tablespoons of water) or place directly in the pot of soup, sauce or meat.

Maximize use of the food processor. Leave it on the counter. You will use it to advantage for puréeing, cutting, grating, or chopping an end piece of cheese, leftover ham, chicken, carrots, celery, onions and other cooking ingredients. Then freeze these ingredients in small bags or sealed plastic containers for later use.

Clean up as you go. Have a large bowl of hot soapy water on hand to wash dishes as you finish using them.

Plan to involve the children. They can wash veggies, assemble a simple recipe, set the table… (see next page).

Have catered food delivered. Some caterers deliver fresh or frozen dishes in portions for two, four, six or eight people. It is often cheaper than a restaurant and the food has been homemade by the caterers!

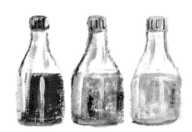

"Help" in the Kitchen!

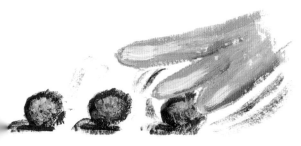

Cooking with your child gives you an opportunity to give her some individualized attention and to ensure some real help…in a few years. It also increases the chances that she will eat her meal (but there is no guarantee).

Moreover, as your child grows up feeling comfortable in the kitchen from the age of six or seven, she is contributing and this builds self-esteem. Here are some things that your child can do in the kitchen:

- Open a can or a box and pour its contents into a bowl.
- Turn the salad spinner.
- Press the buttons on the food processor.
- Measure liquid in a cup.
- Mix ingredients with a spoon.
- Wash firm fruits and veggies (celery, carrots, potatoes, apples) and cut them with a small plastic knife.
- Tear lettuce leaves.
- Arrange bread in a basket.
- Set the table.
- Learn to prepare her lunch box for next day (find recipes and tips in our first book, *Lunch Box*).

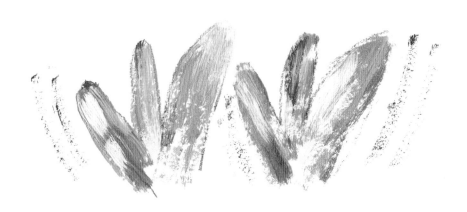

3. Eating According to One's Needs

Do we eat too much or not enough? What should be included in a meal or a snack and in what quantity? Fat and salt: should we or should we not use them? Here are some answers to these questions.

HOW MANY SERVINGS?

What is a serving?

A serving is the quantity of food that produces a measure of nutritional elements. In the same food group, different sized servings of varying foods are nutritionally equal. This means that each food in that group provides approximately the same nutritional elements and can be interchanged.

	1 to 3 years*	3 to 5 years*	6 to 8 years	8 years +
Pasta, rice and potatoes	15 - 45 ml (1-3 Tbsp)	45 - 75 ml (3-5 Tbsp)	75 - 125 ml (5 Tbsp-1/2 cup)	125 ml (1/2 cup)
Bread	1/4 slice	1/2 slice	1 slice	1 slice
Fruit	15 - 45 ml (1-3 Tbsp)	45 - 75 ml (3-5 Tbsp)	75 - 125 ml (5 Tbsp-1/2 cup)	125 ml (1/2 cup)
Vegetables	15 - 45 ml (1-3 Tbsp)	45 - 75 ml (3-5 Tbsp)	75 - 125 ml (5 Tbsp-1/2 cup)	125 ml (1/2 cup)
Milk	60 - 80 ml (4 Tbsp-1/4 cup)	80 - 125 ml (1/4-1/2 cup)	125 - 160 ml (1/2-3/4 cup)	250 ml (1 cup)
Cooked meat poultry and fish	15 - 45 ml (1-3 Tbsp)	30 g (1 oz)	30 - 60 g (1-2 oz)	60 g (2 oz)
Cooked legumes	15 - 45 ml (1-3 Tbsp)	45 - 75 ml (3-5 Tbsp)	75 - 125 ml (5 Tbsp-1/2 cup)	125 ml (1/2 cup)
Eggs	1/4	1/2	3/4	1

* In the preschool years, calculate approximately one tablespoon (15 ml) of food per year of age.

You can refer to these quantities when portioning out servings on your child's plate. It is always preferable to serve small servings first and let your child ask for more. A full plate could discourage him and turn him off before the first mouthful. It is very likely that he will eat more than the minimum indicated on the chart.

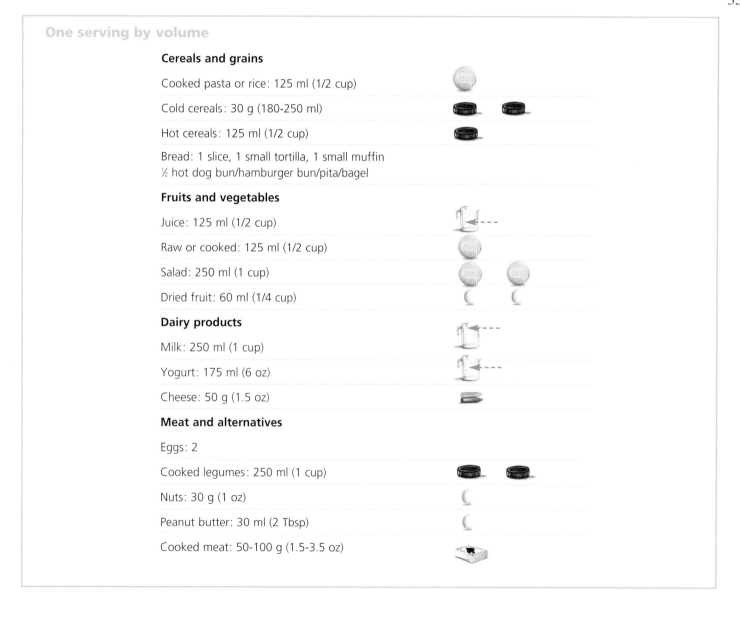

One serving by volume

Cereals and grains

Cooked pasta or rice: 125 ml (1/2 cup)

Cold cereals: 30 g (180-250 ml)

Hot cereals: 125 ml (1/2 cup)

Bread: 1 slice, 1 small tortilla, 1 small muffin
½ hot dog bun/hamburger bun/pita/bagel

Fruits and vegetables

Juice: 125 ml (1/2 cup)

Raw or cooked: 125 ml (1/2 cup)

Salad: 250 ml (1 cup)

Dried fruit: 60 ml (1/4 cup)

Dairy products

Milk: 250 ml (1 cup)

Yogurt: 175 ml (6 oz)

Cheese: 50 g (1.5 oz)

Meat and alternatives

Eggs: 2

Cooked legumes: 250 ml (1 cup)

Nuts: 30 g (1 oz)

Peanut butter: 30 ml (2 Tbsp)

Cooked meat: 50-100 g (1.5-3.5 oz)

How much should we eat?

Most people supply their energy and nutritional needs daily by eating a number of servings from each of the food groups as follows:

36

Cereals and grains:	5 to 12 servings daily
Fruits and vegetables:	5 to 10 servings daily
Dairy products:	2 to 4 servings daily
Meats and alternatives:	2 to 3 servings daily

Can we limit ourselves to the minimum number of servings?

The smaller numbers usually represent the minimum daily requirement of food to supply our nutritional needs, while additional servings satisfy our appetite or energy (or caloric) needs. What is important to remember is that after having consumed the minimum quantity required, we may have achieved our needs from the nutritional point of view (the point at which we can stop worrying!). But we probably will still be hungry. We will then search for additional calories by eating more of one food group (some children will fill up with bread) or other less nutritional foods (butter, oily foods, pastries, or candies).

What if we don't eat the suggested servings?

When we cut back frequently on servings from a particular food group, growth and health can be negatively affected. In reality, there will be days when we will eat less of a food group and others when we will eat more. This is acceptable if the average over a period of two or three weeks stays within the range of the suggested servings from each group. One tip: following dinner, add up the servings consumed during the day and plan to include the missing servings in the following day's menu.

What if a certain food is overeaten?

This is common with children, especially with milk and cereal products, particularly bread. This is not a big deal as long as the average consumption for the other food groups reaches the minimum required. On the other hand, if a child overeats one food group at the expense of others (which could happen, for example, if he drinks lots of milk or juice and is no longer hungry at mealtime) it will be necessary (and only then) to impose some limits because no food group can be substituted for another.

Is it difficult to eat the number of suggested servings?

It is easier than you might think. The reason is simple: a serving is usually much smaller than we imagine. For example, a club sandwich contains three servings of cereals and grains, and one plate of spaghetti easily contains four cereal and grain servings. A large orange juice in the morning equals four servings of fruit. A cup of salad is small by most standard servings. At the restaurant a 300 g (10.5 oz) steak provides enough servings for two days for one person.

What quantity is appropriate?

This depends on several factors, such as size, weight, sex, level of physical exercise and the body's ability to burn calories. It is therefore futile to use appearance or even weight as a base to decide how much or how little one should eat. That's what we did in the 1930s. Statistics on children of all ages (and all adults) show that one person can eat twice as much as another who has the same physical appearance and does the same exercise.

To complicate the picture, body requirements vary not only from one person to another, but according to the year, month and even the day or the meal. A child can stuff herself one day and fast the next. Therefore it is not always easy to know how much she is going to eat at the next meal! But as we have discussed in the first chapter, it is not necessary to know…the child's body (and ours also) knows it. Our second book (*À table, les enfants!*) dealt with this subject in detail.

The "margin of error"

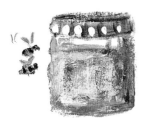

There is a gap between the number of calories necessary to satisfy our nutritional needs and the total calories necessary to fulfill our energy needs. Normally, one-half to two-thirds of the required calories are used by the body's energy needs. Consequently it is not necessary that all food eaten be nutritious. There may be some margin for less desirable choices such as candies and pop. So, if from time to time our child asks for a candy rather than a fruit, don't worry — he will probably have fulfilled his nutritional needs for the day.

WHAT IS A GOOD MEAL?

A meal should supply...

On the plate:

- **A meat or alternative (eggs, legumes, nuts and seeds or their butters).** This group is essential to supply protein and nutrients such as iron and zinc. The proteins contribute to appetite satisfaction and supply (because they also contain fat) the long-term energy necessary to last until the next meal.

- **A starchy food (potato, pasta, spaghetti, rice, bulgur, etc.).** In addition to being nutritious, starchy foods help satisfy your appetite. Note that it is not necessary or even desirable to eat only whole grains. Fiber and other components of whole grains may interfere with iron and zinc absorption. Focus on three servings of whole grains daily. That is already more than most of us consume.

- **Two vegetables or fruits.** By having two vegetables or fruits at each meal we increase the chances that our child will eat at least one! It could be a fruit (canned peaches) and a vegetable (corn), or two vegetables (a salad and tomato sauce in the lasagna) or two fruits (a large fruit salad). Juices, soups and fruit desserts count as well. Do not be afraid to use canned or frozen foods to reduce preparation time, and to serve vegetables with a little butter or sauce to make them more appetizing and satisfying.

Some examples:

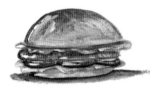

- Hamburger with raw vegetables and tomato juice.
- Roast beef, mashed potatoes, green beans and cabbage salad.
- Fried chicken with vegetables and rice.
- Meat lasagna with salad.
- Hot chicken sandwich with peas and carrots.

On the table:

- **Bread and butter.** Whole grain or white bread is a good "fill up" and a nutritious food which a child turns to when nothing else in his meal appeals to him. Butter or margarine, a concentrated energy source, helps supply a child's need for calories and gives the feeling of fullness (refer to: The Fat and Salt Question, pg 42).

- **Milk.** This is the "official" drink of the meal. Your child should drink 500 ml (2 cups) daily. Milk supplies substantial quantities of protein and is the primary source of calcium and vitamin D for children and adults. Of course our little angel will be more inclined to drink her milk if we set the example. If your child cannot tolerate milk it is better to serve water rather than juice or pop. Above all, don't force a child to drink milk. We offer it and we wait. Occasionally you can flavor it, but be careful: if we try too hard the child will guess your game. He will decode the fact that it must be important for him to have his milk if we go to so much trouble…

For the little ones?

Most children are ready to come to the family table before they are one year old. The same menu will fit the whole family, but we may have to adjust the format, the texture or consistency of some foods to help our children master them. For example:

- Prepare soups that a child can drink or prepare them just thick enough to allow for the use of a spoon.
- Cut food in small bite-sized pieces.
- Cut meat into small pieces.
- Choose ground meat rather than chops or steak.
- Prepare foods that are soft and moist.
- Serve food at room temperature.
- Serve salad without dressing.
- Use a small fork and spoon and childproof dishes.

SNACKS

Most kids cannot go from one meal to the next without a snack. As their needs are great and their stomachs are small, they are simply incapable of consuming enough in a single meal to keep them satisfied until the next. It is better for them to eat small quantities often (about every two to three hours) to give them a continuous supply of energy. It also provides more flexibility to round out their daily needs. This does not imply feeding them cookies and ice cream on demand! Snacks, like meals, should be planned.

The content

An apple or some baby carrots usually will not be sufficient, especially if your child is very hungry or if she has to wait two or three hours before dinner (which is usually the case). To be nourishing, sustaining and filling, snacks must include carbohydrates (fruit, juice, bread, muffins or cereals) and protein (cheese, milk, yogurt, nuts, etc.). The former is quickly digested and provides almost immediate energy for the child. Hunger is appeased for a short period as this energy is provided. The latter carries the child until the next meal by slowly and gradually releasing glucose into the bloodstream.

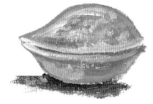

Some examples:

- Fruit pieces with cheese or yogurt.
- Dried fruit with nuts or seeds.
- Cream cheese with crackers.
- Bread or crackers with peanut butter or a glass of milk.
- Dry cereal or biscuits with milk.

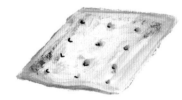

Timing

Snacks must be reasonably spaced between mealtimes. By lunch or dinner the child should be hungry enough to want to eat and to perhaps accept a new food. If the snack is too large and his appetite is reduced at dinner time, it would be advisable to give the child his snack earlier in the afternoon. This way he will pig-out less (as he will have less appetite) and will be more motivated to eat at the next meal. If the time between lunch and dinner is too long, the child could have two snacks. Make the first one more substantial, and this will satisfy him for two or three hours. Later, a small snack (a glass of juice, some raw veggies, a piece of fruit, or two or three crackers) will hold him until dinner.

The place

We should not let our children run or wander about the house with food. As with meals, it is preferable for children to sit down comfortably at the table for their snack, and re-charge before resuming their activities. However, there is nothing wrong with popcorn at the movies occasionally or a glass of juice during the family game of Scrabble.

TOO MUCH LIQUID?

A child who drinks too much liquid, no matter how nourishing it is, will not eat as well at mealtime. It will be more difficult for her to fulfill her needs. The reason is simple: by taking, a large space in the stomach the liquid cuts the appetite for solid foods which are denser in calories and nutrients. Here are some strategies to ensure that your child drinks enough — but not too much.

Milk

Does your child drink more than 500 ml (2 cups) daily? Check that she eats enough food from the other food groups: cereals and grains, fruits and vegetables, and meats and alternatives (refer to the table pg 34). It may be necessary to limit her daily consumption of milk.

Juice

Kids generally like juice and if we let them, they would drink it nonstop. The American Academy of Pediatrics recommends limiting juice consumption to one glass (125-175 ml) (1/2-3/4 cup) a day for children from 1-6 years of age and to 2 glasses (250-375 ml) (1-1 1/2 cups) a day for children from 7-18 years of age. A good tip to reach this goal is to reserve juice for breakfast or snack and have milk at lunch or dinner.

Pop

These are the most popular drinks in North America (well before milk and juice), with a sad average consumption of approximately one can per day per child (along with its 150 calories and 10 teaspoons of sugar). This liquid candy cuts the child's appetite for healthy food and also contains a good number of additives.

Is your child thirsty?

Offer him water. It is an excellent moisturizer and thirst quencher. As for milk and juice, these should be considered foods and eaten along with meals or snacks. Too many children drink lots and lots of juice or pop when they are simply dehydrated and need water.

THE FAT AND SALT QUESTION

Cooking without salt or fat makes it hard to enjoy food. Fat is necessary. It provides essential fatty acids and facilitates the absorption of fat soluble vitamins. As children have large energy needs but small stomachs, this concentrated source of energy provides them the necessary calories for growth. If their meals contain too little fat, they may not be able to eat in amounts sufficient to fulfill their caloric needs. Finally, as fat slows the emptying of the stomach and provides energy over a long period of time, the child will not feel hungry or tire as quickly.

Although it is not advisable to restrict salt and fat too severely, likewise it is not recommended to empty the whole salt shaker in the soup or to use the whole pound of butter in the frying pan! You will use only the amount necessary to enhance the taste of food. Children are naturally very focused on their sense of hunger and of being full (often better than adults), and know when they are no longer hungry. Unless butter, margarine, dressing or any other fatty or salty food becomes a forbidden food (children find them more attractive precisely because they are forbidden) the child may use it generously (for example, spreading butter liberally on toast) only because his little body needs it.

Some suggestions

- Add a moderate amount of salt while cooking (1 ml (1/4 tsp) per cup of food).
- Use canned vegetable if desired.
- Use bacon or very salty food only on occasion.
- Plan for a small amount of fat while cooking (approximately 5-10 ml (1-2 tsp)) per serving.
- Preferably use monounsaturated fats (olive, canola, or peanut oil), and non-hydrogenated margarine, or use butter judiciously.
- Avoid fried foods, chips, and pastries. If your child overeats these bad fat foods, they may take the place of the good fat foods.
- Avoid vegan diets (no egg or dairy products) for children. Plant foods (legumes, vegetables, fruits, cereals and grains) are generally high in fiber but low in fat and thus are low energy foods. As these foods are filling, a child may not be able to consume an adequate amount of food to supply his essential nutrients and fats for energy.

- Cook the same menu with a moderate fat content for the whole family. This will ensure that Mom and Dad will consume a reasonable amount of fat while encouraging a lifetime of healthy eating habits in their children.

- Plan for richer foods in children's menus and then (as always), let them decide what they will eat. By letting the child follow her instincts of hunger and fullness, she will eat more fat when she needs more calories (when very active or during a growth spurt) and less fat when she does not need as much. For example, you could offer her:

  o Homogenized milk at mealtime.
  o A slice of cheese on pasta or rice.
  o A sauce on meat or vegetables.
  o Butter on bread, potatoes or vegetables.
  o Vinaigrette with salad.
  o Ice cream for dessert.
  o Peanut butter on toast at breakfast.
  o Nuts or a slice of cheese for snacks.

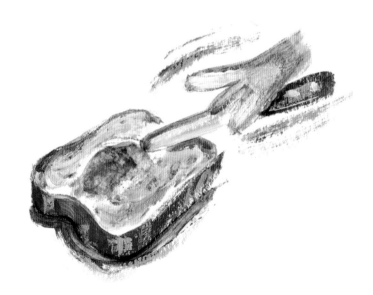

4. Choose Your Foods

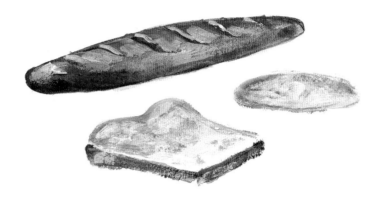

Less saturated fat, trans fat and sugar, not too many calories, more fiber, omega 3, calcium, folic acid…it's not easy finding your way to healthy eating! So here's some easy tips to help you make the right choices when reading labels.

THE BASIC FOOD GROUPS

Grains and cereals

Bread

Ideally, whole wheat flour should be first on the list of ingredients and the only flour used. The label should read "stone ground" which indicates that the wheat has been ground on stone in the ancestral manner, therefore preserving all the nutrition of the original whole grain. Note that "twelve-grain," "bran bread," or "rye bread" are primarily white breads, since white flour (or wheat flour or enriched flour) is the first ingredient listed on the label.

Breakfast cereals

Here again, the words "whole wheat or whole grain" should be the first ingredient on the label. For cereals with little sugar content, choose those with a maximum of 5 g (the equivalent of one teaspoon) per 30 g (1 oz) serving. Note that for cereals containing fruits, you can allow a little more sugar because the quantity listed includes the natural fruit sugar.

Pasta

If you don't choose whole wheat pasta, go for white pasta with the word "enriched" on it. Iron and the B vitamins (thiamine, riboflavin and folic acid) have been added to white pasta to compensate in part for the loss of these nutrients during the refining of the grain.

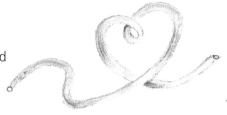

Rice

Brown rice is to rice what whole wheat is to bread: the most nutritious choice. The next choice would be converted white rice (stewed rice). Because of the stewing process, the nutritional elements of the bran and the germ from the heart of the grain are maintained even though they are eliminated in the process. Converted rice is therefore more nutritious than regular white rice or instant rice, but does not pretend to be as good as brown rice.

Crackers

If the product has at most 1 g of trans and saturated fat and 250 mg of sodium per serving of 30 g (1 oz), it is very good. For a superior product check the list of ingredients and see if whole wheat flour (not white flour, enriched flour, wheat flour or unbleached flour) is the only flour listed.

Cakes and muffins

Are there any baked products that consist of anything but sugar, bad fats and calories? Yes, but you have to look for them! They should contain at least 2 g of fiber and no more than 2 g of saturated fat per serving.

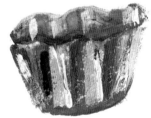

Social tea cookies

Without being nutritional superstars, some cookies are of merit, having a maximum of 2 g of trans and saturated fat per 30 g to 40 g (1 oz to 1.5 oz) serving. Others have an added bonus of 2 g or more of fiber. They provide a wise way to satisfy a sweet craving.

Granola bars

The best are made of whole cereals, nuts and fruits, without too much sugar or trans fats. Three rules to follow when choosing them: at least 2 g of fiber, at most 15 g sugar and 1 g of trans and saturated fat all together per bar.

Fruits and Vegetables

Fresh, frozen or canned

There is nothing like a ripe fruit or vegetable, freshly picked and eaten on the spot! But canned and frozen products are also very good value.

- **Frozen products.** They are blanched and frozen within hours of harvest. There should be no salt, color, preservatives or any other additives. According to several studies, frozen foods can be more nutritious than fresh produce! Avoid buying a frozen product where the food is clumped; use within three months of purchase; and cook without defrosting.

- **Canned foods.** They are picked when ripe and at the top of their nutritional value, and canned within hours of harvest. Their nutritional value remains stable for a year or two and generally compares well with fresh or frozen produce. You can simply reheat vegetables in the preserving liquid which has been brought to the boiling point.

- **Fresh produce.** The quality of fresh fruit and vegetables deteriorates quickly, so buy them very fresh and avoid impulse buying: purchase produce only when you intend to use it within a week.

Fruit juice

The best is made of 100% pure juice with no additional sugar (or sucrose, glucose or fructose), color, or artificial flavor. Do not confuse fruit juice with fruit punch, fruit cocktail, or sparkling fruit beverages, which are generally full of sugar or diluted with water. From a nutritional standpoint, orange juice is number one, followed by grapefruit, grape and pineapple juices. Note: nothing equals a fruit freshly juiced like homemade orange juice or the non-processed apple juice (brown in color) sold in grocery stores. However, reconstituted products from concentrates (like frozen juice), are quite acceptable.

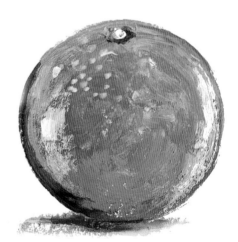

Vegetable and cocktail juices

250 ml of these vegetable juices are the equivalent of 2 servings of vegetables.
They contain only 40-60 calories. Their one drawback: salt, unless you buy those varieties with reduced sodium content. Note: some products fill 100% of our daily needs of Vitamin C, while others supply only 5%. Read labels carefully!

Canned fruit

Whether you prefer fruit in chunks or puréed, it is best to use a "no sugar added" or "in own juice" type. With all the new products in the grocery stores we now have choices beyond the old reliable apple sauce.

Dairy Products

Milk

All types of milk (skim, 1%, 2% or homogenized) have the same nutritional value. For children under two it is best to use homogenized milk (3.25%). The fat from the milk remains a significant source of energy and essential fatty acids (especially for the brain), for babies and toddlers whose growth is rapid and stomach small. Homogenized is fine up to five years of age. You could switch to partly skimmed (1% or 2%) from the age of two if your child loves to drink milk, his growth is normal and his meals include other forms of fat (oil used in meal preparation, meat, cheese, ice cream, butter or margarine, vinaigrette). Skim milk is to be avoided until the age of five.

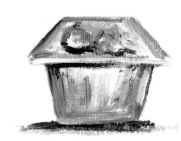

Yogurt

Ideally, it should not contain more than 1.5% fat ("% M.F." on the label), no aspartame (there are still doubts as to the harmlessness of this artificial sweetener) and at least 18% of the daily calcium requirements per 175 g (6 oz) serving. There is no shortage of choices on the market.

Yogurt with "Probiotics"?

In the dairy section we now find a new generation of yogurt with probiotics. The word probiotic, meaning "for life," are living bacteria, which, when consumed in sufficient quantity, are beneficial to your health. These good bacteria, especially those in yogurt, can help prevent diarrhea, constipation and bloating. Scientists believe that probiotics may stimulate the immune system, prevent colon cancer and reduce cholesterol. Of course not all probiotics are equal. Each culture offers different benefits. Activia yogurt by Danone, for example, contains the active culture Bifidobacterium DN-173 010 (also known under the name BL™), which has been clinically proven to be effective. The daily consumption of one Activia yogurt can improve intestinal "transit" significantly and therefore the regularity and healthy functioning of the digestive system.

Cheese

Calcium and protein without excessive saturated fat and salt? The best choice would be cheese with 18% fat ("% M.F.") or less. Processed cheeses, cheese spreads or slices which are high in salt are best avoided.

Meat and Alternatives

Fresh meat and poultry

We prefer lean meat cuts such as rump, fillet, round steak, sirloin and skinless poultry. It is best to choose lean or extra lean ground meat, especially if you do not plan on draining the cooking fat before adding other recipe ingredients (meat loaf or spaghetti sauce, for example).

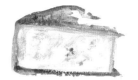

Seasoned meats and poultry

Meat such as chicken breast, pork souvlaki and other seasoned, precut and processed foods are convenient. Some brands are low fat, but the price we pay is a product high in sodium since they are generally immersed in seasoned salt brine (which adds weight to the meat) or they are coated with highly salted sauces.

Breaded fish and poultry

Be cautious with fried and heavily breaded meat products. The best choice is 3 g of saturated fat (or 9 g total fat) and up to 500 mg sodium per 100 g (3.5 oz) of cooked meat or 120 g (4 oz) of raw meat.

Deli foods

They contain more fat, salt and additives and less protein than fresh meat. Preferably choose items that have 800 mg of sodium and 5 g of fat or less per 100 g (3.5 oz) serving. Tip: limit a serving to 2-3 slim slices (about 60 g) and leave room for tomato and cucumber slices, as well as lettuce.

Legumes and tofu

These meat alternatives bring a good deal of protein and little fat to your meal. Legumes are high in fiber. Sliced regular tofu (firm or soft) plain or seasoned, is a perfect choice for soups, prepared dishes and stir-fried vegetables. Choose tofu products containing calcium sulfate: one 100 g (3.5 oz) serving can supply as much calcium as two glasses of milk!

Oils and Fats

Vegetable oil

Due to their richness in good unsaturated fat, olive, canola, and soy oils are presently praised by all experts. You can use olive oil for its flavor in vinaigrettes and canola for a more neutral taste in cooking. Note that cold pressed versions are better from a taste and nutrition point of view. However, as they do not take heat very well, you should use them for vinaigrettes and light cooking (pan fried), rather than for deep-fried cooking.

Margarine

The best margarines do not have more than 0.5 g trans and saturated fat per 10 g (2 tsp) serving. They are soft and non-hydrogenated. Tip: assess the composition of the finished product rather than the oils used, as the manufacturing process changes the quality of the original oils.

PREPARED FOODS

Frozen meals

These meals rarely feed as many people as indicated on the package. If you refer to the nutrition label, this means that we absorb generally more saturated fat and sodium than estimated by the manufacturer. These items generally contain high amounts of starch (pasta, rice or potatoes) and few vegetables. It is best to have them with a good soup, vegetable juice, salad or raw veggies if we want a nutritious meal. The best frozen meals have 5 g saturated fat (or 15 g total fat) and 800 g of sodium or less per serving (between 150 and 275 g [5 oz and 9 oz] of the cooked product).

Frozen pizza

No perfection here! Too much saturated fat and sodium…unless you restrict yourself to the very small serving often suggested on the packaging (but who would be satisfied with 1/6 of a pizza?). The best option is to be happy with a modest serving (1/4-1/3 of the pizza) and satisfy the balance of your appetite with a large serving of salad or raw veggies. Our healthy guideline: a maximum of 5 g saturated fat (or 15 g total fats) and 800 mg sodium per serving of 1/3 of a 25 cm (10 inch) diameter pizza.

Spaghetti sauce

The problem with canned sauces is their high salt content. You can also criticize the high fat content in meat, cheese and especially creamed varieties of sauces (alfredo, cream, or rose). The healthy choices: 800 g of sodium and 2 g of saturated fat or less per 250 mg serving.

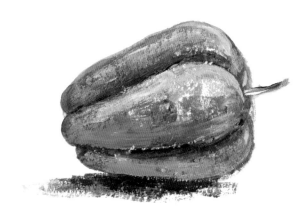

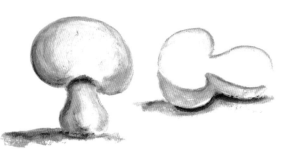

Canned soups

Salt has always been the negative ingredient in canned soups. The percentage of fat should not be neglected, especially in creamed soups (clam chowders, cream of mushroom, cream of chicken, etc). The best soups should have, at most, 500 g sodium and 3 g of fat per 250 ml (1 cup) serving.

Frozen desserts

If you love these delicious desserts you should choose light ice creams, frozen yogurts or sherbets and select versions with 8 g of fat or less per 250 ml (1 cup) serving.

Chips and other salted snacks

None of these are good for you. However, some are not as bad as others…they should contain a maximum of 200 mg sodium and a total of 3 g trans and saturated fat per serving of 30 g (1 oz).

BEVERAGES

Bottled water

Heavy users of bottled water and those who must restrict their input of sodium should choose a product "without sodium." This is the case for most spring water.

Flavored carbonated water

These are naturally flavored lemon, lime or orange sparkling waters, or with some additional juice (the percentage of juice is specified on the label). They are thirst quenching but you should select those without added sugar.

Carbonated beverages

This liquid candy (such as colas) comes with a large dose of additives, caffeine, and phosphoric acid, which promote the growth of kidney stones. If you drink too much caffeinated beverages this may decrease your sleep and increase your stress levels. The diet version? They are not healthy but they have the advantage of being sugar-free and have practically no calories.

Spritzers

These sparkling drinks are made of fruit juices (the percentage is often indicated on the packaging) and carbonated water. Some have the advantage of containing neither added sugar nor coloring, but consist simply of juice added to carbonated water, with natural flavoring. They are not to be confused with pop.

Sport beverages

They are quickly absorbed sugar fuels and replace the water and minerals (like sodium, potassium and calories) lost in body sweat. They can be helpful during prolonged exercise (more than 2 hours) but are not really necessary. An athlete does not need added flavors or artificial colors.

Malt beverages

These Ovaltine-type mixtures are made of a base of barley, cocoa and skim milk powder, with the addition of several nutrients including iron. You add hot or cold milk, stir, and enjoy in small sips. A pleasant way to drink your daily calcium!

Drinkable yogurts

They are drinkable, can easily be carried, and provide a nice change from juice or milk in the lunch box. Usually they are without added flavor, artificial color, and they are made of yogurt with real fruit added (puréed or concentrate). The better ones do not have more than 1.5% fat and no less than 25% of the daily value of calcium per 250 ml (1 cup) serving, which is as much as milk.

Flavored milks

These drinks contain protein, calcium and vitamin D…the same desirable nutrients in milk. However, they have added sugar, sometimes a lot of sugar. Healthy choices should contain 20 g of sugar at most and 1.5 g of saturated fat per 250 ml (1 cup) serving.

Soy beverages

The enriched versions generally supply all the nutrients found in milk (calcium, riboflavin, vitamin B12, vitamin A and D) in addition to vitamin C, iron, folic acid and other desirable nutrients. Protein in soy helps protect your heart, as does the omega 3 fat and fiber, if it is added (the label will inform you). Soy beverages contain no lactose. The best choices: no more than 20 g of sugar and 1.5 g of saturated fat per 250 ml (1 cup) serving.

Coffee

Three or four cups a day of regular coffee is a small and harmless pleasure, if cream, sugar, chocolate or whipped cream are not added. If these are added, these can become as rich as milkshakes.

Tea

This natural drink, with no artificial flavor, color, or other additives is the most consumed beverage in the world (after water)! Green or black, tea has the same caffeine content, which is 2-3 times less than coffee. Daily consumption of 2-5 cups is associated with a lower risk of cardiovascular diseases and cancer. The only negative is that the tannin in tea encapsulates iron from food and prevents it from being absorbed. Rather than drinking tea during meals, wait at least two hours or plan to have a good source of vitamin C at mealtime to neutralize the effects of the tannin.

Ice teas

Commercial ice teas usually do not contain coloring or artificial flavor. They are prepared with real infused tea to which sugar is added (but less than soda pop) or an artificial sweetener.

Herb teas

These are infusions of dried plants other than teas (Camellia sinensis). They do have valuable properties: lemon balm tea, lime blossom tea, orange blossom and chamomile tea promote relaxation, while mint, rosemary, sage, verbena and chamomile teas facilitate digestion. Herb teas contain no sugar or caffeine.

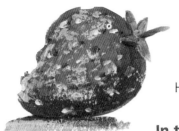

OUR FAVORITE FOOD PRODUCTS

Healthy and practical, they make life easier.

In the Freezer
Frozen fruit

Some frozen fruits are individually frozen and sold wrapped in ziplock bags. There is no need to defrost them. They go directly from the bag into your pancake mix, fruit crisp, ice cream, fruit juice, yogurt, milkshakes and exotic drinks. For a snack or a fast dessert they can be served as is (frozen) in a dessert cup, or you could use them in a yogurt or chocolate sauce. Let them melt in your mouth…

Frozen vegetables

There is no waste here. Only the edible part has been packaged and you need only remove what you want. The balance can be kept in the freezer for up to a year. This is a good reason to keep a variety of frozen vegetables. Already washed, cut and even assorted (Asian, Mexican and Californian mixes, etc.), they can be put in the microwave for a few minutes, in the skillet, in the steamer, or added directly to soup, rice cooking water or pasta in the final minutes of cooking.

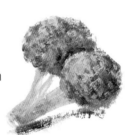

Light frozen desserts

There is nothing like iced milk or yogurt, sherbet, or "light" ice cream for an impromptu dessert: ice cream with coulis or fruit, peach melba, filled crepes (try commercially made Crêpes Bretonne), ice cream sandwiches, or fruit milkshakes. The best contain 8 g of fat or less per 250 ml (1 cup) serving.

Concentrated fruit juice

It can be kept for months. Nutritionally, it compares well with refrigerated juices. Since it has been concentrated by evaporating the part that is water, it takes very little room in the freezer. Concentrated juice can be used to season rice cooking water and marinades for poultry and pork. It can also be used to enhance (without adding fat or salt) the taste of sweet potatoes or carrots and pan-fried vegetables and chicken. The products "with calcium" can help increase your source of this important nutrient.

Frozen fruit bars

The commercial variety prepared with juice and puréed fruit are incomparably better than the usual popsicles made with sugar, flavor and colored water.

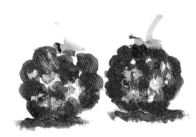

Wonton wrappers

These wrappers can be used to easily create delicious little morsels! You fill their center with chicken, ham, roast beef or shrimp (an opportunity to use leftovers) and you fold to shape triangles and seal with egg white. Oil lightly and cook in the oven for 10 minutes on each side, then enjoy with sour cream or salsa. Other suggestions: boil them for 2 minutes and serve the Chinese way with a bouillon and diced vegetables, or incorporate a peanut butter sauce to create a delicious hot main course.

Boneless turkey or chicken breasts

The white meat of poultry is extra lean. Adults and children love white meat, whether it's breasts, cubed and sautéed, in kabobs, barbequed on the grill or broiled in the oven. A tip to speed recipe preparation: before freezing, cut the fillets or breasts according to their planned use and put the pieces, well labeled, in freezer bags or plastic containers.

Frozen turkey

A 7 kilo (15 lb) turkey gives about 2.5 kilo (5.5 lb) cooked meat. This is enough to prepare several dishes (pâtés, hot sandwiches, rice dishes, etc.). Once cooked, let the poultry cool before deboning it, then freeze slices and pieces in servings sufficient for a family meal. This way you will always have a basic ingredient on hand for a soup, salad or any recipe requiring a cooked meat.

Cooked shellfish

There are shrimp, crab, lobster, and for less money and practically no fat, products made from arctic char or whiting with added crab or lobster flavor. Already prepared, cooked and flaked or formed in rolls, they can replace the same quantity of chicken or beef in your favorite recipes, or added as is to pasta dishes, chowders, salads and sandwiches. The small rolls are also excellent appetizers served with a dip or vinaigrette.

Individually frozen fish fillets

A real catch! Fillets of sole, haddock, arctic char or salmon are individually frozen, then vacuum packed to keep their freshness and facilitate separation. You can use one or two fillets and keep the others in the freezer for later. They are ideal for a chowder, a rice dish, kabobs, steamed as is or cooked in the microwave oven on a few minutes for one, two or several people.

Grated cheese in ziplock bags

A small quantity can do a lot to enhance flavor, especially when using a cheese that has a strong flavor such as parmesan, swiss, old cheddar or gruyère. Use only the quantity necessary. Put leftovers in the freezer and make sure to extract as much air as possible from the bag. Grated cheese is very handy for soups, hamburgers, sandwiches, omelets, pizzas, salads, lasagna and for all cheese-topped dishes.

Stuffed pasta (ravioli, tortellini)

They keep easily for three months in the freezer, cook rapidly, and can be accompanied by any sauce. The challenge is which one to pick!

In The Refrigerator

Natural yogurt

This is a nice way to get your calcium and maintain a healthy level of intestinal flora. Use it for dips (mixed with grated veggies, salsa, a little chopped garlic, herbs, Dijon mustard, or sundried tomatoes), vinaigrettes, marinades, cold sauces, or poultry, white meat or fish. At dessert time it is also delicious with chunks of fruit, granola cereal or as a garnish for waffles, pancakes and cakes.

Pasteurized liquid eggs

Who said you can't make an omelet without breaking an egg? These liquid eggs are sold in handy 250 ml (1 cup) cartons (about 5 large eggs). They contain 80% less cholesterol and fat than regular eggs and are composed of fresh eggs and other natural ingredients. They prepare and taste just like regular eggs. Because they are pasteurized, they can be used in drinks, mayonnaise, homemade ice cream and other items not requiring cooking.

Chopped nuts

Almonds, hazelnuts, peanuts and other nuts are full of good unsaturated fat and proteins and provide long-lasting energy. They also add crunch and an exotic touch to sandwich fillings, yogurts, morning cereals, casseroles, fruit or vegetable salads and baked products (cookies, muffins, crisps, cakes). Because of their oil content, however, they can become rancid. It is best to keep them in the refrigerator for 4-6 months, or even in the freezer up to one year rather than in the storage pantry.

Flax seeds

Thanks to their fiber content and good omega 3 fatty acids, flax seeds help protect against diabetes, cardiac diseases, cancer, intestinal and inflammatory problems, as well as menstrual and menopause symptoms. Nothing is better! Grind at the last minute and incorporate in your morning cereals, yogurts, apple sauce, vinaigrettes, hamburger meat and baked products. Whole flax seeds can be kept for a year at room temperature and up to a month in a refrigerator when already ground.

Prewashed baby spinach

No need to trim or wash them several times to get rid of grit. This good vegetable is ready to go. Fresh or cooked, as a salad or an accompanying vegetable (pan fry or braise in the microwave before seasoning with a little balsamic vinegar) or in prepared meals (lasagna, soups, fettuccini, white or tomato sauces, pizza, sandwiches, potatoes, stuffing for chicken breasts, or veal stuffing, meat loaves and frittatas).

Prewashed salads

These are colorful tender greens ready to eat. You need only add a garnish and dressing. The use of ziplock bags allow you to use only the necessary quantity for each prepared salad.

Hummus

This is a chick pea purée to be used as a dip for raw veggies, chips, or as a spread on bread or crackers.

Pesto

This vibrant, colorful sauce, full of flavor, can be used as a marinade or to coat chicken, pork or salmon, or used as a spread for sandwiches and pizza. It can also be added to mashed potatoes, yogurt dip, soups, pastas, tomato or your favorite cream sauce. For long-term storage, freeze in ice cube trays. When the cubes are frozen, transfer them to freezer bags.

Salsa

Only 15 calories per 30 ml (2 Tbsp) serving, salsa is great with nachos, tacos and fajitas. Nothing can compare to this Mexican ketchup as a garnish for hamburgers, sandwiches, baked potatoes, scrambled eggs or frittatas. Equally, it can be used as a sauce, marinade or a quick vinaigrette for pizza, kernel corn, bean salads, kabobs or grilled chicken or pork.

Fresh skimmed cheese

This is a good alternative to sour cream, mayonnaise or cream cheese, all of which are very rich. Eat it simply on its own or with herbs or grated vegetables, as a spread, a dip, or to stuff cannelloni. Incorporate sundried tomatoes, salsa, olives or chopped nuts as a canapé garnish.

In the Pantry

Canned fish in water or stock

They contain a good deal of protein, omega 3 fatty acids and calcium (when the bones are used in the recipe) and are low in calories and saturated fat. Open the can, drain and add to pizza, tacos, spaghetti sauce, lasagna, bruschetta and salads. They can be deep fried, added to pasta or rice dishes, or even used as a filling for sandwiches or as a garnish on canapés.

Grilled soy nuts

These are good to cook or as a snack. They are soy beans cooked in oil. They are ideal for children who have allergies to peanuts, for school snacks and are nutritious.

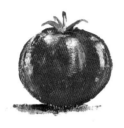

Canned tomatoes

This is a wonderful base for soups, salsa, chili, meat and macaroni sauce, stews and casseroles. They are sold with only salt, sugar and additives, or pre-seasoned, but you can add your own touch (onions, garlic, herbs, hot peppers, pesto and leftover vegetables) by puréeing them in a food processor for a smooth texture. Try it as a sauce for chicken or braised pork.

Round flatbread

Garnish and place in the oven. This is an opportunity to use your leftover vegetables, cooked meat and cheese… Or fruit — spread a little jam or coulis, fruit chunks and grated chocolate, grill for 5 minutes and dessert is served! As a quick appetizer, spread the flatbread with a little bruschetta, flavored oil, sundried tomatoes or basil pesto, sprinkle with parmesan cheese, grill and cut into triangles or rectangles, and serve. Flatbreads freeze well.

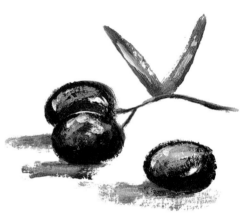

Enriched cream of wheat

One serving of 45 ml (3 Tbsp) of dry cream of wheat supplies half the recommended daily intake of iron. It's very easy to incorporate into food (hamburger meat, soups, vegetable purées, omelets, casseroles and baked items).

Dried fruit

Cranberries, raisins, dates, apricots and prunes are natural candies which can be consumed as is or rehydrated (in water, juice or alcohol). They are great as snacks or as an addition to morning cereal. They are used for meat and poultry sauces, stuffing, rice, fruit salads, yogurts, apple sauce, muffins, cookies and cakes. Also use dried fruit as a quick fuel injection to keep in your purse or the glove compartment of the car…just in case!

Silken tofu in Tetra Paks

It can be kept several months without refrigeration. It whips well and is incognito in soups, cream sauces, spreads, desserts, and whipped drinks.

Bananas

They are used for a great number of recipes (muffins, cakes, donuts, banana bread, etc.) but can also be enjoyed as a popsicle (peel and freeze on a stick and serve with or without chocolate sauce), in fruit salad, dips, fondue, or cooked in parchment paper 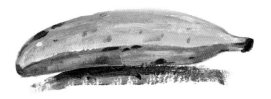 in the oven for 10-15 minutes (garnish first with a little honey, butter and chopped nuts). Too ripe? Just freeze them as is (in their skin) in anticipation of recipes to come.

Canned sliced peaches

They are delicious when garnished with granola, yogurt, ice cream, on your morning cereal, or in homemade fruit salads and compotes. They can be made into coulis for iced desserts and cakes. They are used for pie, cake, pudding and fruit square recipes. Why not dice and add to chopped meats (pork, beef, lamb) and the accompanying sauce.

Unsweetened apple sauce

It is particularly appreciated as a snack in the lunch box. It can be used as an alternative to oil in your muffin and cake recipes. It is a quick sauce for pork chops, kabobs, cakes, morning waffles and cereal.

Bouillon cubes, or canned stock (light in sodium)

This gives added flavor with little fat. You can cook rice in it or incorporate it into mashed potatoes, or use it to sauté meat or vegetables. It can also be used as stock for Chinese stir-fries (add a little red wine, bay leaf or garlic powder to taste) which can then be re-used as a base for soup. For a quick meat, poultry or vegetable sauce, dissolve 2 tablespoons (30 g) of corn starch in 300 ml (1.2 cups) of stock, and simmer until thick, stirring constantly.

Canned condensed cream soups (light in fat)

You can reconstitute it with milk rather than water, and add a little leftover cheese, tofu, poultry or cooked beans to make a light and satisfying meal. Diluted with a little water or milk, it also makes a creamy sauce, meat loaf, scalloped potatoes, rice or pasta dishes.

Soup mixes

Rice, barley, lentils and beans…it's all there! You need only add water or stock, your favorite herb and let it simmer until cooked. Soup is served!

Canned legumes

They have excellent nutritional value. There is no need to soak them or simmer for a long time. Open the can, rinse with running water (to eliminate excess salt) and they can quickly be added to fajitas, chilies, rice, stuffings, soups, salads, pasta sauce, stews and casseroles. They can also be blended with yogurt or salsa for a dip or sandwich filling.

Baked beans in tomato sauce

A serving of 250 ml (1 cup) provides 14 g of fiber, the equivalent of seven slices of whole wheat bread. In addition to being low in fat, it is also very, very economical. All you do is open, pour and reheat.

Date and fig cookies

Their main ingredient is dates or figs. They satisfy your sweet tooth, and supply more iron, potassium and fiber than most commercial cookies.

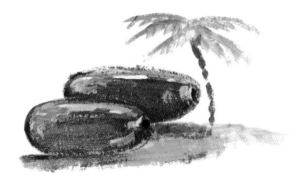

Recipes

Basic Recipes
and Accompaniments

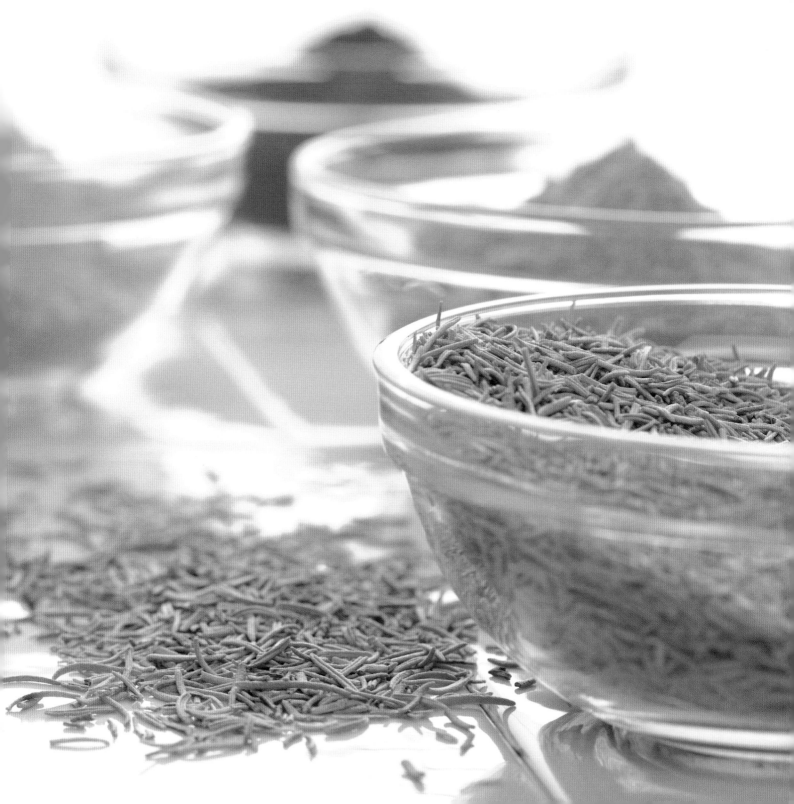

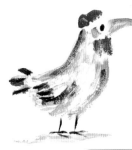

Basic Chicken Stock

Your soups will never be the same after using homemade chicken stock.

Preparation: 5 min Cooking time: 1 h 30 Makes 2 l (8 cups)   **Can be frozen**

1	large quartered chicken 2-3 kg (4-6 lb)
	or 4 chicken legs with bones
2	large carrots, rough cut
1	large onion, quartered
6	garlic cloves, unpeeled
	celery leaves
1	bay leaf
10	peppercorns
	coarse salt

Place the quartered chicken in a large saucepan. Pour in cold water to cover the chicken. Add the vegetables and seasonings. Bring to the boil on high heat. Skim any foam off the surface. Reduce heat to medium and let simmer one hour, loosely covered, skimming if necessary.

Take out the chicken and remove bones. Reserve the flesh and dispose of the carcass and skin.

Meanwhile, continue cooking the stock for about 20 minutes. Strain into a bowl. Throw out the vegetables.

Refrigerate the stock for at least 2 hours and remove the solidified fat from the surface. The stock will keep refrigerated for 2 days or frozen for 6 months.

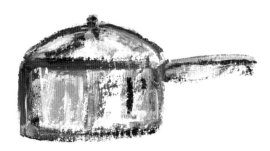

TIP
To insure that all ingredients remain submerged, place the top part of the steamer on the surface. This will also make skimming the stock easier.

VARIATION
For a "chicken noodle soup" that resembles a commercial soup, add turmeric (this gives a lovely golden color to the stock), some vermicelli, slivered chicken and a bit of fresh parsley.

Cream of Corn Soup

This soup filled with vegetables, can be puréed and served creamed.

15 ml	(1 Tbsp)	oil
1/2 pkg	(750 ml/3 cups)	soup vegetables packaged prepared vegetables*
500 ml	(2 cups)	frozen kernel corn
45 ml	(3 Tbsp)	flour
500 ml	(2 cups)	hot vegetable or chicken stock
1 can	(385 ml/14 oz)	evaporated milk
1 pinch		pinch nutmeg
		salt and pepper

* Fresh prepared vegetable mixtures, found in the refrigerated section of your grocery store, are very versatile. A mix of carrots, celery, cabbage, onion and turnip can be added to soups, stews and spaghetti sauce.

In a large saucepan, heat the oil on medium. Add the vegetables and corn. Cook for 10 minutes or just until the vegetables are soft.

Sprinkle the flour on the vegetables, mix well and cook a few more minutes.

Stir in the hot stock and the evaporated milk, stirring constantly until thickened.

Add a pinch of nutmeg. Salt and pepper to taste. Lower the heat and simmer gently for 5 more minutes.

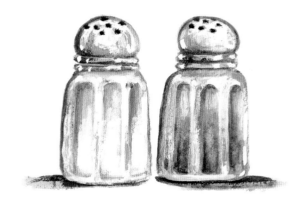

TIP
- Self-adhesive labels and a permanent felt pen are very practical to identify and date cooked items.

VARIATION
- Add cooked shrimp or crab meat and replace the nutmeg with fennel seeds.

Roasted Root Vegetables

Slip these into the oven and prepare the rest of the meal during the roasting period.

Preparation: 15 min Baking time: 30 min Servings: 6

4		large carrots, peeled
4		potatoes, peeled
2		parsnips or white turnips, peeled
30 ml	(2 Tbsp)	oil
7 ml	(1 1/2 tsp)	salt
30 ml	(2 Tbsp)	chopped fresh chives or 10 ml (2 tsp) dried chives

Preheat the oven to 230°C (450°F).

Cut the carrots into strips lengthwise. Place in a large bowl. Stir in the oil, salt and chives.

Spread prepared vegetables evenly on a large baking sheet lined with parchment paper. Cook 30 minutes or until the vegetables are golden.

Serve as an accompaniment to Piccata Turkey (pg 126), Tomato Pesto Pork Cutlets (pg 106) or Meat Loaf (pg 128).

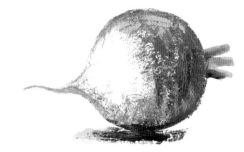

TIP

- Place your wooden or plastic chopping board on a damp tea towel to keep it from slipping.

VARIATIONS

- To vary the flavor: when the vegetables are roasted stir in grilled chopped nuts, blue cheese or crumbled feta, curry paste, or either lemon or orange zest.
- Replace the oil, salt and chives with a mix of 45 ml (3 Tbsp) honey, 15 ml (1 Tbsp) lemon juice and 15 ml (1 Tbsp) oil. Salt to taste.
- Do not restrict yourself to only the suggested vegetables: make your own combinations. Example: sliced winter squash, sliced beets and onion rings. The method is the same and the cooking time is about 20 minutes.
- Eat the roasted vegetables with rice or cooked barley, salt and pepper; add a little chopped parsley and you have roasted vegetable pilaf!

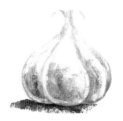

Ratatouille

This savory preparation lends itself to multiple uses and freezes well.

15 ml	(1 Tbsp)	oil
1		fennel bulb, cubed
2		onions, coarsely chopped
2		red and/or yellow peppers, diced
4		garlic cloves, slivered
5 ml	(1 tsp)	fennel seeds
2		zucchini, diced
6		tomatoes, chopped coarsely or 1 can (540 ml / 19 oz) diced tomatoes
		salt and pepper
50 ml	(1/4 cup)	chopped fresh basil

Preheat the oven to 180°C (350°F).

In an ovenproof thick-bottomed saucepan, heat the oil on medium. Fry the fennel, onion and peppers, stirring from time to time for 10 minutes or just until the vegetables are slightly golden.

Add the garlic and fennel seeds and mix. Cook about 1 minute or just until the mixture smells savory.

Add the zucchini and tomatoes. Add salt and pepper. Cover and roast for 45 minutes or until vegetables are tender and ratatouille is slightly thickened. Stir in the basil before serving.

Serve with Potato Frittata (pg 164) or Tuna Croque-Monsieur (pg 131). This could also be used to prepare Tortellini with Ratatouille Sauce (pg 149) or Chicken Cacciatore (pg 113).

TIPS

- Fast meal : cover the bottom of individual ramekins with hot ratatouille. Make an indentation and crack an egg into this nest, being careful not to break the yolk. Cook in a preheated oven 200°C (400°F) for 8-10 minutes or until the eggs are soft cooked (they continue to cook in the hot ratatouille). Serve with crusty bread.

- Fast meal : fry 500 g (1 lb) ground beef in a large frying pan until done. Add 750 ml (3 cups) ratatouille and 1 can (213 ml / 7 _ oz) tomato sauce. Heat well and stir in about 1.5 L (6 cups) macaroni-type pasta of your choice. Serve with parmesan and a green salad.

VARIATION

- For a traditional flavor, replace the fennel bulb with cubed eggplant cooked along with the zucchini.

Tomato and Cucumber Salad

This salad will bring texture and freshness to Crispy Tofu (pg 153) and to main courses of fish, beef or grilled chicken.

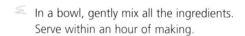

Preparation: 10 min Servings: 4

2		tomatoes, diced
1/2		English cucumber, peeled and diced
1		green onion, chopped
45 ml	(3 Tbsp)	fresh parsley, chopped
30 ml	(2 Tbsp)	oil
15 ml	(1 Tbsp)	wine vinegar
		salt and pepper

In a bowl, gently mix all the ingredients.
Serve within an hour of making.

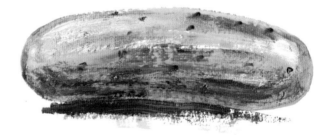

VARIATIONS
Note: for these variations double the amounts of parsley, oil and wine vinegar.

- Niçoise Salad: add a can of flaked tuna and some black olives and replace the wine vinegar with 30 ml (2 Tbsp) lemon juice. Serve on thinly sliced romaine lettuce.

- Moroccan Salad: add 1/2 can (540 ml / 19 oz) well rinsed and drained chick peas, and 5 ml (1 tsp) ground cumin. Serve on a nest of couscous.

- Italian Salad: add 1/2 can (540 ml / 19 oz) white beans, rinsed and drained. Replace the cucumber with a small fennel bulb, chopped into bite-sized pieces and add 15 ml (1 Tbsp) tomato pesto. Serve mixed with cooked pasta.

- Mexican Salad: add 1/2 can (540 ml / 19 oz) black beans, rinsed and drained well, 250 ml (1 cup) kernel corn and 15 ml (1 Tbsp) chili powder. Serve with cooked white rice.

Garlic and Mint Yogurt Sauce

Veggies have never had it so good...

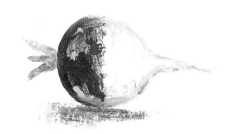

1		garlic clove
1 ml	(1/4 tsp)	salt
125 ml	(1/2 cup)	plain yogurt
2 ml	(1/2 tsp)	dry mint or 7 ml (1 1/2 tsp) fresh chopped mint
		salt and pepper

Crush garlic in a mortar or with the blade of a large knife on the cutting board and mix with salt to form a purée. Stir the mint into the yogurt. Salt and pepper to taste.

Serve this as an accompaniment to East Indian Chick Peas (pg 156) or Moroccan Style Pitas (pg 88).

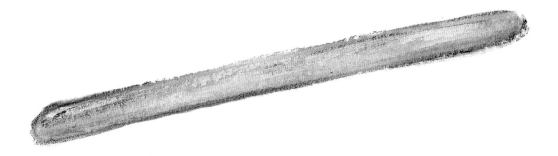

TIPS
- Use this sauce as a marinade for whole or cubed boned chicken breasts. Put the sauce with the chicken in a plastic bag, close and shake well to coat the chicken, then place in the refrigerator or freezer.
- To remove the odor of garlic on your fingers, wet your hands and rub them on the stainless steel tap or sink.

VARIATIONS
- Tzatziki version: add 50 ml (1/2 cup) peeled, seeded cucumber, finely grated and well drained.
- Raita version: double the quantity of yogurt and add 125 ml (1/2 cup) peeled and finely grated cucumber, 125 ml (1/2 cup) finely chopped tomatoes and a large pinch of cumin. Delicious with grilled chicken.

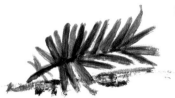

Tomato Sauce

This basic sauce can be used in the preparation of lasagna, spaghetti or Parmesan Chicken (pg 122) or Chicken on Fennel (pg 117).

Preparation: 5 min Cooking time: 50 min Makes 1,75 l (7 cups)   **Can be frozen**

30 ml	(2 Tbsp)	oil
6		garlic cloves, slightly crushed
3 cans	(796 ml /28 oz)	diced plum tomatoes
10 ml	(2 tsp)	coarse salt
50 ml	(1/4 cup)	fresh chopped basil
5 ml	(1 tsp)	dried oregano

In a large saucepan, heat oil on medium and sauté garlic for 2 minutes or until lightly golden.

Add the tomatoes and salt. Bring to the boil. Lower the heat and simmer, stirring occasionally for 45 minutes or until thick.

Stir in the basil and oregano. Using a whisk or food processor, make a smooth purée, if desired.

MY CHILD CAN...

- Tear whole tomatoes up with her fingers. She will love it!

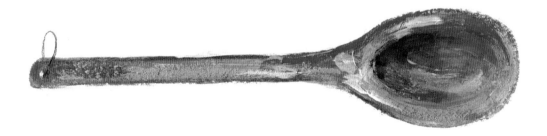

TIPS

- Double the recipe and freeze it in family or individual portions.
- For an improvised meat sauce stir leftovers from Meat Loaf (pg 128) into the tomato sauce.

White Sauce

This white sauce differs from the traditional béchamel. Even without the fat, this rich sauce goes well with lasagna, macaroni and cheese or the preparation of any pasta recipe.

Preparation: 5 min Cooking time: 5 min Makes 500 ml (2 cups)

500 ml	(2 cups)	milk
75 ml	(1/3 cup)	flour
2 ml	(1/2 tsp)	salt
		pepper

In a saucepan, heat the milk with the flour while stirring constantly until thick, about 3 minutes.

Add salt and pepper to taste.

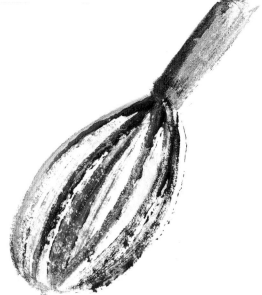

VARIATIONS

- Cheese sauce: stir 125 ml (1/2 cup) grated old cheddar cheese or grated parmesan and a pinch of dry mustard powder into the thickened sauce.
- Rose sauce: stir 15 ml (1 Tbsp) tomato paste and a large pinch of dried oregano into the thickened sauce.
- Florentine sauce: stir 125 ml (1/2 cup) defrosted, well-drained spinach along with a pinch of nutmeg into the thickened sauce.

Vegetable Variations

Vegetables should be a part of each meal and, prepared as we suggest, will receive high marks!

GRILLED VEGETABLES

Preparation: 10 min Baking time: 10 min Servings: 5

Preheat broiler. Mix 3 chopped garlic cloves with 45 ml (3 Tbsp) oil. Salt and pepper to taste. Cut into quarters, 2 peppers, 2 zucchini, 2 plum tomatoes and 2 onions, and brush the surfaces with oil. Place on a parchment-lined baking sheet. Grill under the broiler for 10 minutes or until vegetables are golden.

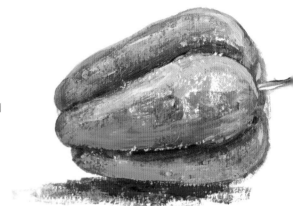

FENNEL SALAD

Preparation: 10 min Servings: 4

Thinly slice a small fennel bulb, a small red onion and an unpeeled red apple.
Sprinkle all with 15 ml (1 Tbsp) olive oil and 10 ml (2 Tbsp) balsamic vinegar. Salt and pepper to taste.

CARROT RIBBONS

Preparation: 10 min Cooking time: 5 min Servings: 4

Using a vegetable peeler or a mandolin, make long ribbons to the heart of 2 carrots. Place in a steamer and steam 5 minutes or until al dente. Place on a small serving platter. Sprinkle with 10 ml (2 tsp) lemon juice and 5 ml (1 tsp) oil, then dust with 15 ml (1 Tbsp) chopped fresh chives. Salt and pepper to taste.

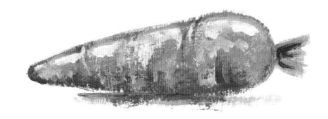

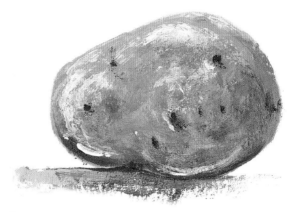

SALTED POTATOES

Preparation: 5 min Baking time: 30 min Servings: 4

Use sufficient oil to generously coat mini potatoes. Sprinkle with coarse salt. Spread on a parchment-lined baking sheet. In an oven preheated to 230°C (450°F) bake the potatoes for 30 minutes or until they are tender and golden. For a different look, use a mix of white, red and blue mini potatoes. They can be bought prepackaged.

POTATOES AND SAUSAGE

Preparation: 5 min Baking time: 30 min Servings: 4

In an oven preheated to 230°C (450°F), cook mini potatoes with 3 unpeeled garlic cloves, a few fresh rosemary sprigs, in an enameled, earthenware or pyrex dish for 30 minutes, along with 6 veal or turkey sausages, pricked several times. Just before serving, cut the sausages on the diagonal and fingerpress the garlic cloves, and dispose of the peel (use the flesh to spread on crusty bread slices).

GRILLED TOMATOES

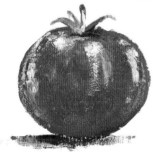

Preparation: 10 min Baking time: 20 min Servings: 4

Preheat oven to 200°C (400°F). Place 8 tomato halves in an ovenproof casserole dish. In a small bowl, mix 45 ml (3 Tbsp) grated parmesan, 30 ml (2 Tbsp) bread crumbs, 15 ml (1 Tbsp) oil and 5 ml (1 tsp) dried basil or oregano. Place approximately 10 ml (2 tsp) of this mixture on each tomato half. Pepper to taste. Bake the tomatoes for 20 minutes or until tender.

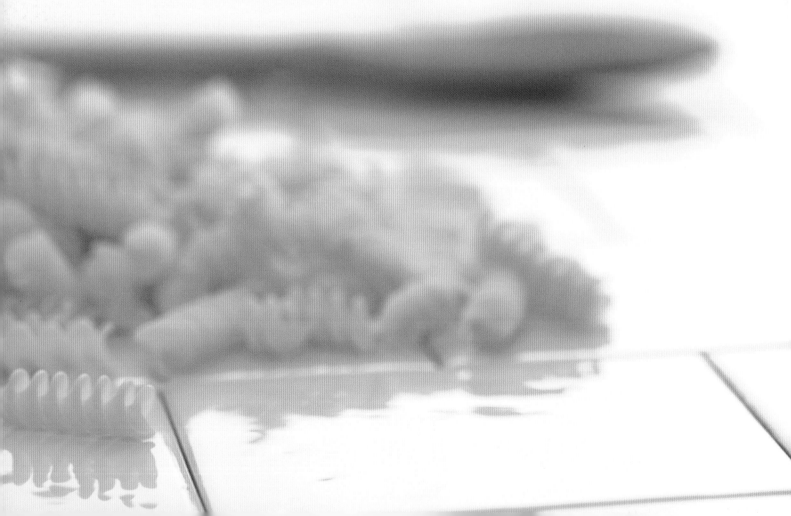

Main
Courses

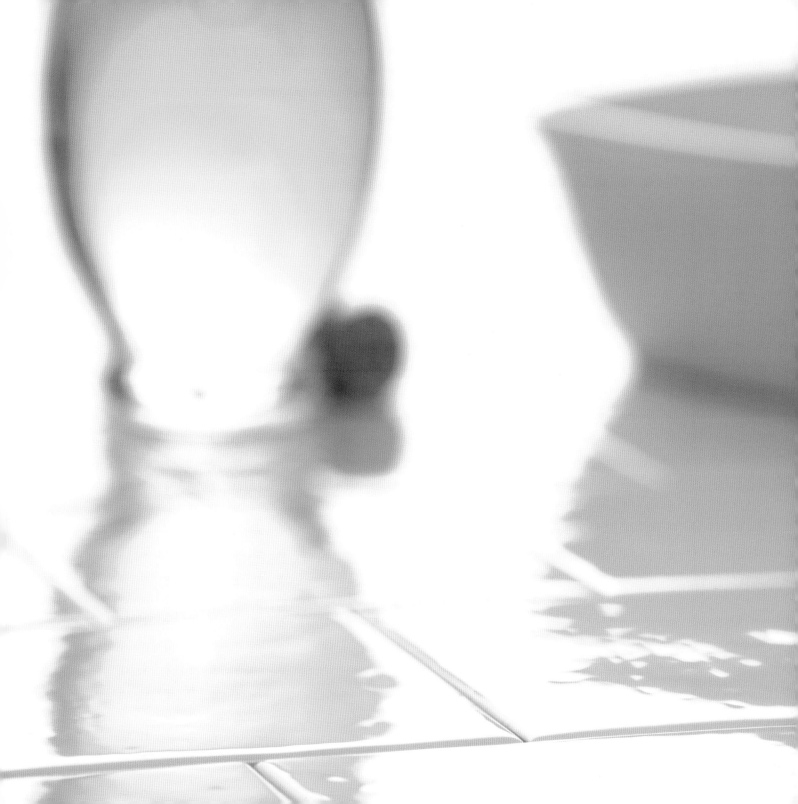

Main Courses ~

Soups

Pasta and Chick Pea Soup – Pasta e ceci

Did you know that 125 ml (1/2 cup) chick peas provide as much iron as 90 g (3 oz) cooked ground beef? And, they are succulent!

Preparation: 10 min Cooking time: 20 min Servings: 4

**Vegetarian
Can be frozen**

10 ml	(2 tsp)	oil
2		garlic cloves, chopped
1		sprig fresh rosemary or 7 ml (1½ tsp) dried crushed rosemary
1 can	(540 ml/19 oz)	diced tomatoes
500 ml	(2 cups)	beef or vegetable stock
250 ml	(1 cup)	water
1 can	(540 ml/19 oz)	chick peas, rinsed and drained
125 ml	(1/2 cup)	raw macaroni (or other short pasta)
		salt and pepper
60 ml	(4 Tbsp)	grated parmesan

In a large saucepan, heat the oil on medium and sauté garlic and rosemary for 30 seconds or until the garlic is golden. Add the tomatoes, stock and water and bring to the boil.

Meanwhile, crush approximately 250 ml (1 cup) chick peas with a potato masher. Mix the crushed chick peas, whole chick peas and macaroni into the stock and tomato mixture. Salt and pepper to taste.

Remove the rosemary sprig. Simmer the soup, uncovered, for 10 minutes or until the pasta is cooked.

Sprinkle 15 ml (1 Tbsp) parmesan on each bowl of soup and serve.

MY CHILD CAN...

- Crush the chick peas.

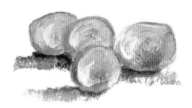

TIPS

- If this soup is reheated the next day, add some stock or water as it will have thickened.

- Before beginning a recipe, read it in its entirety to avoid any surprises (waiting time, ingredients needed).

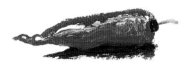

Asian Tofu Soup

A hearty meal in a bowl!

Preparation: 10 min   Cooking time: 15 min   Servings: 5   **Vegetarian**
(MARINATE 15 MIN)

45 ml	(3 Tbsp)	soy sauce
15 ml	(1 Tbsp)	honey
2		garlic cloves, finely chopped
1 pkg	(454 g/16 oz)	firm tofu, cut in 2 cm (3/4") cubes
1.5 L	(6 cups)	chicken or vegetable stock
45 ml	(3 Tbsp)	fresh, finely chopped ginger
500 ml	(2 cups)	julienned frozen green beans
1 pkg	(120 g/4 oz)	Chinese rice noodles
4		green onions, cut on the diagonal
		toasted sesame oil (optional)
		sauce aux piments hot sauce (optional)

In a bowl, mix soy sauce, honey and garlic. Add cubed tofu to the mixture, coating well. Let this marinate while preparing the stock. (You could also let the tofu marinate 24 hours.)

In a large saucepan, bring stock and ginger to the boil. Stir in green beans, the tofu cubes and marinade. Bring back to the boil and add the noodles. Cook 5 minutes or until noodles are done.

When serving, separate the vegetables and share them equally in the bottom of each soup bowl and gently pour the hot stock over this. Garnish with sliced green onions. Add a few drops of toasted sesame oil and hot sauce if desired.

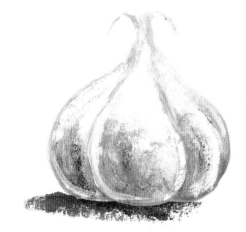

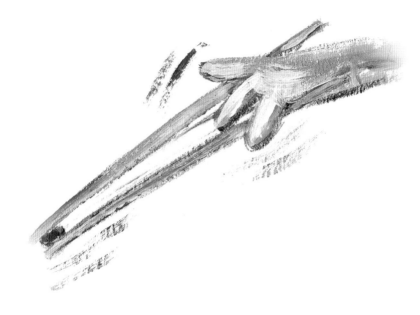

MY CHILD CAN...

- Cube the tofu.
- Prepare the marinade and coat the tofu.
- Learn how to use chopsticks.

TIP

- Break the noodles in two before cooking them.
  These will be easier to serve and eat, especially for children.

VARIATIONS

- Replace the tofu with cooked chicken or shrimp. For an even more authentic Asian flavor, add tender center stalks of lemon grass, finely chopped, at the same time as the ginger in the stock; garnish soup bowls with a little finely sliced chili pepper rather than the hot sauce.

- If you don't have Chinese rice noodles on hand, use angel hair or vermicelli; cook them al dente according to package instructions.

- You could replace the soy sauce with nuoc mam. This is a clear, highly salted fish sauce used to enhance the flavor of the other ingredients, not to give a fish flavor. There is also a Thai version called nam pla.

Indian Lentil Soup

For typical East Indian flavor, garnish this soup with chopped fresh cilantro when serving.

Preparation: 5 min   Cooking time: 15 min   Servings: 3   **Vegetarian**
Can be frozen

5 ml	(1 tsp)	oil
1		small onion, finely chopped
10 ml	(2 tsp)	curry
1 can	(540 ml/19 oz)	lentils, rinsed and drained
1 can	(398 ml/14 oz)	chicken or vegetable stock
375 ml	(1 1/2 cup)	water
3		thin lemon slices

In a saucepan, heat oil on medium-high. Add onion and cook 5 minutes or until soft. Add the curry and stir until it takes on a pungent aroma.

Stir in the lentils, stock and water and let simmer 10 minutes or until lentils are tender. Purée in a food processor. When serving, place a thin slice of lemon on the soup's surface.

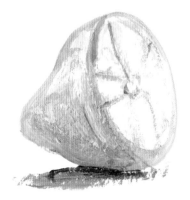

TIPS

- For incomparable flavor, crush the slice of lemon on the bottom of the soup bowl with the back of a spoon.
- Serve a crusty papadum (if you can find a source) with the soup.
  This bread resembles a pita, but has a texture comparable to a cracker.

VARIATION

- Serve this soup with roasted pitas: separate 4 pitas in half, brush them with a mixture of 45 ml (3 Tbsp) olive oil and 5 ml (1 tsp) powdered coriander, then sprinkle with 5 ml (1 tsp) mustard seed. Bake in a preheated oven 180°C (350°F) for 10-12 minutes or until the pitas are golden and crusty. Break the pitas into bite-sized pieces.

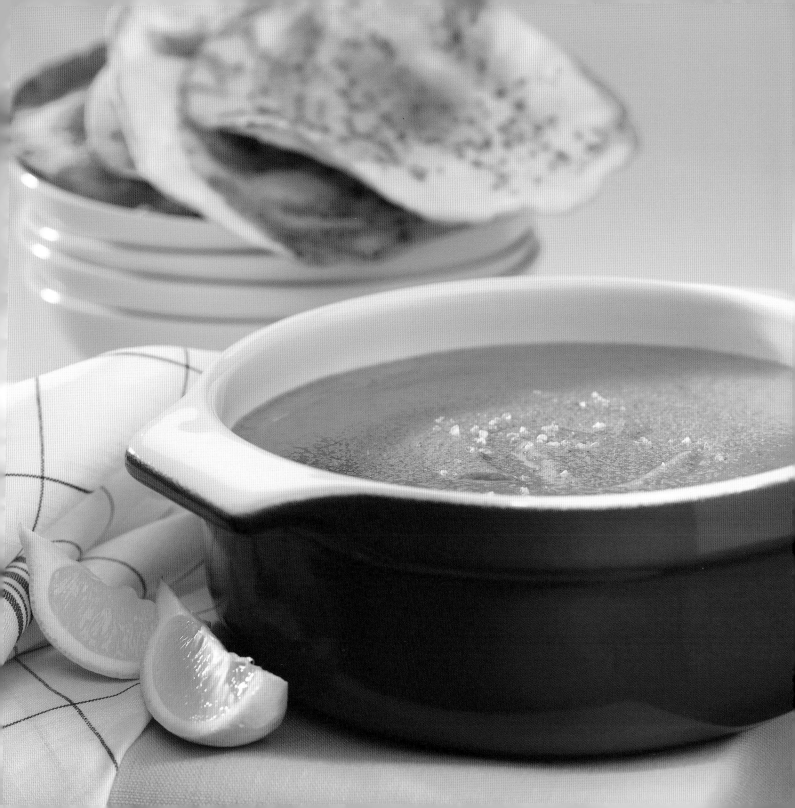

Chicken Rice Soup

The favorite of large and small folk! The addition of turmeric adds a lovely golden color to the stock.

Preparation: 5 min Cooking time: 40 min Servings: 10 **Can be frozen**

2.5 l	(10 cups)	chicken stock (commercial, or see pg 64)
500 g	(1 lb)	skinless chicken breasts
1 pkg	(700 g/25 oz)	soup vegetables*
250 ml	(1 cup)	long grain brown rice
5 ml	(1 tsp)	salt
5 ml	(1 tsp)	turmeric
50 ml	(1/4 cup)	fresh chopped parsley
		pepper

* Fresh prepared vegetable mixtures, found in the refrigerated section of the grocery store, are very versatile. A mix of carrots, celery, cabbage, onion and turnip can be added to soups, stews and spaghetti sauce.

In a large saucepan, pour in the stock and poach the chicken on medium for 20 minutes (or 30 minutes if frozen chicken is used). Remove the poached chicken and set aside.

Add the vegetables, rice and salt to the stock. Bring to the boil, lower heat and simmer, partially covered, 20 minutes or until vegetables and rice are cooked.

Cut the chicken into bite-sized portions and add to the soup. Stir in the turmeric and parsley. Pepper to taste and serve.

MY CHILD CAN...

* Cube the cooked chicken.

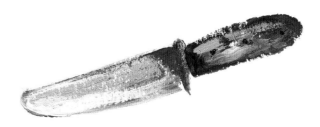

VARIATIONS

* To shorten the preparation, use leftover cooked chicken or a purchased barbeque chicken and low-sodium commercial stock.

* You can prepare chicken in this manner for a salad or chicken sandwiches.

* Treat fresh herb bundles like a bouquet of flowers: place the bundle in a cup or vase containing an inch or so of water to partly cover the stalks, then loosely cover all with a plastic bag to maintain freshness, and refrigerate for up to 2 weeks.

Chicken and Bean Soup

A robust hot meal for a cold winter's night.

10 ml	(2 tsp)	oil
500 ml	(2 cups)	sliced leeks
250 ml	(1 cup)	grated carrots
2 ml	(1/2 tsp)	dried sage
500 ml	(2 cups)	chicken stock
500 ml	(2 cups)	water
1 can	(540 ml/19 oz)	white beans, rinsed and drained
500 ml	(2 cups)	cooked chicken, slivered
2 ml	(1/2 tsp)	lemon zest
		salt and pepper

In a large saucepan, heat oil on medium high. Sauté leeks and carrots for 5 minutes or until cooked.

Add sage and cook until the mixture smells savory. Pour in stock and water and bring mixture to the boil.

Add carrots, beans, chicken and lemon zest and bring back to a simmer. Add salt and pepper to taste and serve.

MY CHILD CAN...

- Grate the carrots.
- Rinse the white beans.

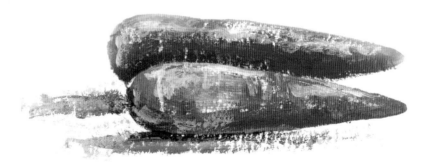

TIP

- For a fast version, use prepared leeks and carrots which are washed and cut up, and a barbequed chicken.

Italian Sausage Soup

Get two birds with one stone! Double or even triple this recipe and freeze in individual servings.

Preparation: 15 min   Cooking time: 30 min   Servings: 6   Can be frozen

400 g	(14 oz)	Italian sausage
15 ml	(1 Tbsp)	oil
1		bulb fennel, slivered or 2 diced celery stalks
1		carrot cut in rounds
1		onion, diced
2		garlic cloves, chopped
500 ml	(2 cups)	chicken stock
500 ml	(2 cups)	water
1 can	(540 ml/19 oz)	diced tomatoes
2 ml	(1/2 tsp)	fennel seed
200 ml	(3/4 cup)	short pasta (tubetti, fusilli, macaroni)
30 ml	(2 Tbsp)	fresh chopped parsley or 10 ml (2 tsp) dried parsley
		salt and pepper
		grated parmesan

Remove the stuffing from the sausage (throw away the casing). In a large saucepan, heat oil on low and fry the sausage meat 5 minutes or until it is well browned. If you wish to maintain the sausage in circles for the soup, cook the sausage whole and then cut it in 1 cm (1/2") rounds. Remove the meat from the saucepan and pour off the fat if necessary.

In the same saucepan, cook the fennel, carrot, onion and garlic for 10 minutes or until vegetables are tender.

Add the sausage to the saucepan, add stock, water, tomatoes and fennel seeds, and bring to the boil.

Stir in the noodles and return to the boil, then simmer 8 minutes or until noodles are cooked. Add parsley, salt and pepper to taste and serve with grated parmesan.

MY CHILD CAN...

- Have fun by removing the sausage stuffing.

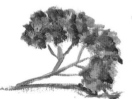

TIPS

- In order to accelerate soup preparation, slice vegetables (fennel or celery, carrots and onion) in the food processor.
- For an even faster preparation, replace the celery, carrots and onion in the recipe with 1/2 package of precut vegetables. The flavor may vary.

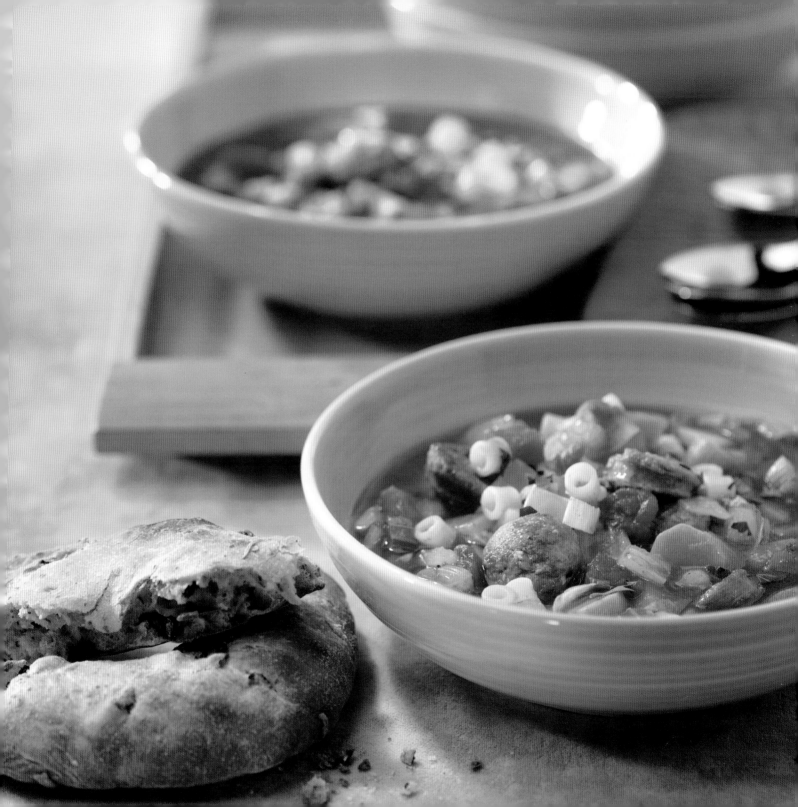

Beef

Parmesan Meatballs

1, 2, 3... here come the meatballs...4, 5, 6...there they go!

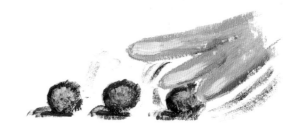

500 g	(1 lb)	ground beef
1		egg
45 ml	(3 Tbsp)	bread crumbs
75 ml	(1/3 cup)	parmesan
50 ml	(1/4 cup)	fresh chopped parsley
		salt and pepper
15 ml	(1 Tbsp)	oil
15 ml	(1 Tbsp)	butter

In a bowl, mix all ingredients thoroughly except oil and butter.

Form ping-pong-sized meatballs (rub some olive oil on hands to facilitate the process). This makes approximately 20-25 meatballs.

In a large skillet, heat the oil and butter on high and sear the meatballs for 15 minutes or until browned, turning often.

MY CHILD CAN...

- Mix the meat and form the meatballs with his hands.

TIP

- Double or triple this recipe and place the quantity needed per meal in freezer bags. Remove the maximum amount of air from the bags before freezing. With the aid of a straw, suck out the air, then close the bag while rapidly pulling out the straw.

VARIATIONS

- Oven baked: place the meatballs on a baking sheet. Bake in a preheated 190°C (375°F) oven for 15 minutes. Serve on a nest of rice accompanied by a spinach salad.
- Spaghetti and meatballs: leave the cooked meatballs in the skillet and add 1 L (4 cups) tomato sauce (commercial or see pg 70); let simmer for 5 minutes and serve on spaghetti noodles.
- Soup: form very small meatballs and cook them in simmering beef stock; add chopped spinach and garnish with parmesan. Serve with crusty bread.

Moroccan Style Pitas

Eat with your fingers, everyone's allowed!

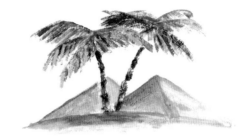

Preparation: 5 min Cooking time: 25 min Servings: 6   **Can be frozen**

125 ml	(1/2 cup)	pine nuts
10 ml	(2 tsp)	oil
1		large diced onion
500 g	(1 lb)	ground beef
15 ml	(1 Tbsp)	cumin
2 ml	(1/2 tsp)	ground coriander
1 ml	(1/4 tsp)	ground cinnamon
2 ml	(1/2 tsp)	salt
1 can	(398 ml/14 oz)	diced tomatoes
6		20 cm (8") diameter pitas, halved
GARNISH		shredded lettuce and plain yogurt to taste

In a small skillet, toast the pine nuts while shaking the pan from time to time, for approximately 3 minutes or until they are lightly toasted. Set aside.

In a large skillet, heat the oil and fry the onion for 3 minutes or until soft. Add the ground beef and brown it while breaking it up into small pieces.

Add the cumin, coriander, cinnamon, salt and tomatoes with their juice. Bring to the boil, lower the heat, and simmer uncovered for 15 minutes or until most of the liquid has evaporated. Stir in the grilled pine nuts. This makes enough to stuff 12 pita halves.

Fill the pita halves with the mixture, garnish with shredded lettuce and yogurt, and enjoy.

MY CHILD CAN...

- Fill her own pita and eat it with her fingers!

TIPS

- Double this recipe and freeze the remaining meat filling.
- Before beginning the cooking, assemble all the ingredients and utensils to be used.

VARIATIONS

- Use the meat filling to make tortilla wraps.
- Serve the meat filling on a nest of basmati rice.

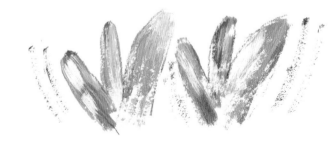

Sage Beef Stew

This stew freezes well in individual or family servings.

15 ml	(3 tsp)	oil
800 g	(1 3/4 lb)	cubed beef
2		large onions, slivered
1 can	(398 ml/14 oz)	diced tomatoes
125 ml	(1/2 cup)	red wine or beef stock
2 ml	(1/2 tsp)	ground sage or 10 ml (2 tsp) fresh chopped sage
		salt and pepper

Preheat oven to 180°C (350°F).

In a large ovenproof saucepan, heat 5 ml (1 tsp) oil. Sear half the cubed beef until browned.

Set the browned meat aside. Add 5 ml (1 tsp) more oil and sear the remaining cubed beef. Keep the seared beef warm.

In the same saucepan, heat the remaining oil and fry the onions until golden. Add the tomatoes, wine and sage. Add the seared beef cubes.
Salt and pepper to taste and mix well.

Bake 1 hour. Serve with mashed potatoes.

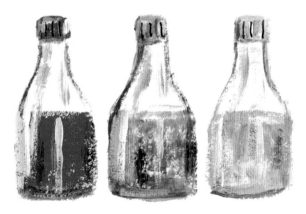

TIPS

- The mashed potatoes can be prepared up to 2 hours in advance. You can avoid the mashed potato top from drying out by coating with milk. Keep warm. Just before serving, stir in the milk, giving a creamier dish.

- Cook small quantities of cubed beef, searing it well, and avoid boiling it in its own juices.

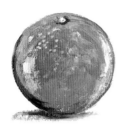

Orange Beef Stir-Fry

The key to success in stir-frying: have all the ingredients prepared and on hand just at the moment of cooking.

Preparation: 15 min Cooking time: 15 min Servings: 6

200 ml	(3/4 cup)	orange juice
45 ml	(3 Tbsp)	hoisin sauce
15 ml	(1 Tbsp)	corn starch
15 ml	(3 tsp)	sesame oil
500 g	(1 lb)	sirloin beef strips
2		chopped garlic cloves
30 ml	(2 Tbsp)	fresh chopped ginger
750 ml	(3 cups)	broccoli flowerets, or approximately ½ of 500 g pkg frozen broccoli
75 ml	(1/3 cup)	water
1		red or yellow bell pepper cut in strips
6		green onions cut into 2.5 cm (1") slices

- In a bowl, mix the orange juice, hoisin sauce and corn starch. Set aside.

- In a wok or large skillet, heat 5 ml (1 tsp) oil on high. Add half the beef and cook 2 minutes or until no pink color remains. Repeat the process with the remaining beef in 5 ml (1 tsp) oil. Keep warm.

- Heat the remaining 5 ml (1 tsp) oil. Add the garlic and ginger and cook 30 seconds or until the mixture smells savory. Stir in the broccoli and water.

- Cover and cook, stirring from time to time, 2 minutes or until the broccoli is sizzling.

- Stir in the reserved hoisin sauce mixture, peppers, and green onion. Bring to the boil while stirring for 1 minute or until the sauce thickens. Stir in the reserved meat. Heat well.

- Serve with steamed basmati rice and a sprinkle of sesame seeds.

TIP
- To achieve fluffy rice, rinse well under running water until the water runs clear before cooking; then sauté in seasoned oil until each grain is coated. Add the water next; calculate 375 ml (1 1/2 cups) liquid for 250 ml (1 cup) raw rice. Cover and let simmer 20 minutes or until the liquid is absorbed.

VARIATIONS
- Replace beef with raw shelled shrimp, and proceed in the same manner.
- Replace the broccoli with 2 sliced zucchini and a package of 227 g (8 oz) quartered mushrooms.

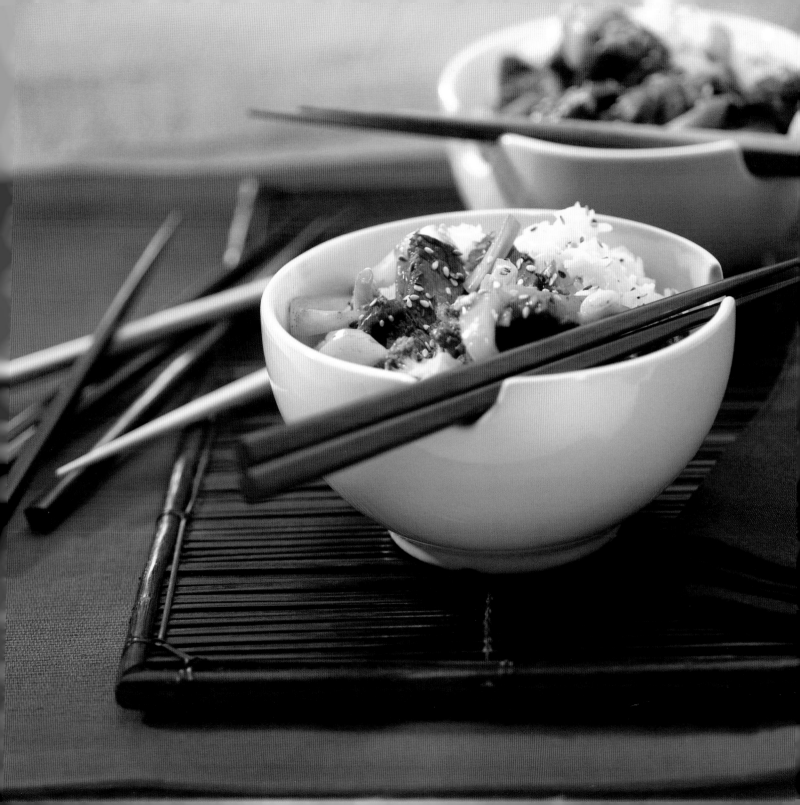

Grilled Beef Flank

Delicious grilled on the barbeque or in a cast iron pan.

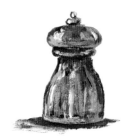

Preparation: 10 min Cooking time: 15 min Servings: 4
(MARINATE 4 H)

30 ml	(2 Tbsp)	red wine vinegar
15 ml	(1 Tbsp)	oil
2		slivered garlic cloves
10 ml	(2 tsp)	dried oregano
5 ml	(1 tsp)	cumin
1 ml	(1/4 tsp)	fresh ground black pepper
1 ml	(1/4 tsp)	cayenne
2 ml	(1/2 tsp)	ground coriander
500 g	(1 lb)	flank beef steak

In a small bowl, mix the vinegar, oil, garlic and spices to form a paste. Rub this paste on all sides of the flank steak. Place on a plate, cover and marinate in the refrigerator for at least 4 hours or overnight.

On an oiled barbeque grill, cook the steak on high for 8 minutes each side. Let it rest 5 minutes and then slice, cutting against the grain of the meat.

Serve with Salted Potatoes (pg 73) and Grilled Tomatoes (pg 73).

MY CHILD CAN...

- Mix the spices and rub the paste into the meat.

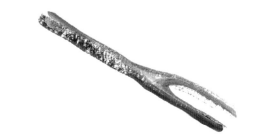

TIPS

- Flank steak has an incomparable flavor but you could substitute inside round fast fry steak.
- A cast iron pan is excellent to cook this steak because cast iron holds and distributes heat well and the surface is anti-stick. Is your cast iron pan gathering dust? It must be seasoned: oil the exterior and interior of the pan and place in a preheated 150°C (300°F) oven for 1 hour, clean it by rubbing with coarse salt with a paper towel and wipe well. If, in spite of this procedure it rusts a bit, season it once again.

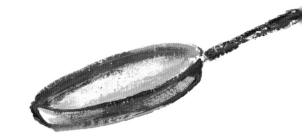

Bolognaise Sauce

This sauce need not be cooked a long time to render it savory. Adding milk to the sauce may seem unusual, but it is the traditional preparation of this recipe in Northern Italy.

15 ml	(1 Tbsp)	oil
2		chopped garlic cloves
2		large onions, diced
1		small carrot, diced
2		bay leaves
1		rosemary sprig or 5 ml (1 tsp) dried rosemary
		salt and pepper
1 kg	(2 lb)	ground beef
250 ml	(1 cup)	red wine or beef stock
1 can	(156 ml/5 1/2 oz)	tomato paste
250 ml	(1 cup)	water
250 ml	(1 cup)	milk

In a large thick-bottomed skillet, heat the oil and sauté the garlic, onion and carrot for 10 minutes or until the vegetables are tender.

Add the bay leaf and rosemary, salt and pepper to taste. Add the ground beef and cook until it has lost its pink color.

Add the wine or beef stock and let simmer 10 minutes or until most of the liquid has evaporated.

Stir in the tomato paste and water. Simmer 15 minutes or until the water has almost evaporated.

Add the milk and simmer 15 minutes more or until the milk has almost evaporated. This sauce is particularly suited to serving with tagliatelli noodles, cooked al dente and garnished with parmesan.

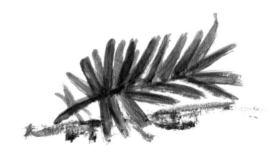

TIP

- When only two teaspoons of tomato sauce are required, what do you do with the remainder of the can? A practical suggestion: line an ice cube tray with plastic wrap and fill the cavities with tomato paste. Place in the freezer, and once frozen, remove the frozen tomato cubes and store in a freezer bag. They will keep up to 6 months in the freezer. You can also buy tomato paste in a tube and use only the amount required.

Steak with Mushroom~Coffee Sauce

A simple preparation with mouth-watering results!

Preparation: 10 min Cooking time: 15 min Servings: 4

2 ml	(1/2 tsp)	cumin
2 ml	(1/2 tsp)	ground coriander
1 ml	(1/4 tsp)	salt
		pepper
15 ml	(3 tsp)	oil
500 g	(1 lb)	beef sirloin steak 1-2 cm (1/2-3/4") thick
1 pkg	(227 g/8 oz)	fresh mushrooms, quartered
4		green onions cut into 1 cm (1/2") slices
3		slivered garlic cloves
5 ml	(1 tsp)	brown sugar
125 ml	(1/2 cup)	hot coffee
45 ml	(3 Tbsp)	balsamic vinegar

In a small bowl, mix the cumin, coriander and salt. Add pepper to taste. Rub the steak with this blend. Set aside.

In a large skillet, preferably cast iron, heat 10 ml (2 tsp) oil on medium heat. Cook the steak to desired degree of doneness or approximately 3 minutes each side. Transfer the cooked steak to a platter, cover and let it rest.

In the same skillet, add the remaining oil and cook the mushrooms and green onions 3 minutes or until tender.

Add the slivered garlic and brown sugar and cook 1 minute while stirring. Add the coffee, balsamic vinegar and meat juices which have accumulated on the platter. Cook the sauce for 3 minutes, reducing it to intensify the flavor. Pepper to taste.

Meanwhile, cut the steak into thin slices, cutting against the grain of the meat. Return the slices to the skillet and reheat in the sauce.

Serve with fried potatoes and/or Roasted Root Vegetables (pg 66).

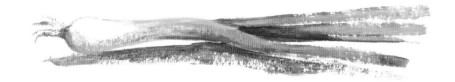

- Mix the cumin, coriander, salt and pepper.
- Rub both sides of the steak with this mixture.

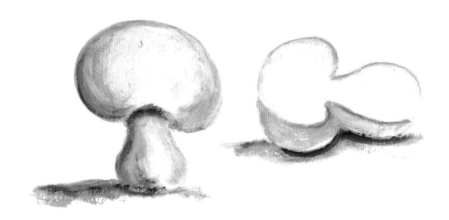

TIPS

- A sharp knife is less dangerous than a dull one. With a dull knife, it is necessary to exert more pressure on the blade and you risk it slipping. To avoid a dull blade, don't soak in water, and only cut on a wood or polyethylene (plastic) cutting board; forget glass, granite or metal.
- Sear meat to seal in the juices and to enhance the flavor. It is seared when it detaches easily from the skillet, then turn it. If it sticks or tears when you go to turn it, it isn't seared sufficiently.
- You can wash the mushrooms in water rather than dry wiping them. It is faster and the dampness will evaporate while cooking.

VARIATIONS

- For a spicier version, add cayenne to the spice mix.
- For a more sophisticated presentation, serve the meat and mushrooms on a nest of spinach or watercress.

Tex~Mex Tacos

A fast and delicious way to include black beans in our diet.

Preparation: 5 min Cooking time: 20 min Servings: 8

Can be frozen

10 ml	(2 tsp)	oil
500 g	(1 lb)	ground beef
15 ml	(1 Tbsp)	chili powder
5 ml	(1 tsp)	dried oregano
2 ml	(1/2 tsp)	cayenne
1		red bell pepper, diced
250 ml	(1 cup)	frozen kernel corn
1 can	(540 ml/19 oz)	black beans, rinsed and drained
250 ml	(1 cup)	water
8		20 cm (8") tortillas
GARNISH		grated cheese, slices of tomatoes, avocados, shredded lettuce, plain yogurt

In a large skillet, heat the oil on medium, sear the meat with the chili and oregano while breaking it up with a wooden spoon.

Add the remaining ingredients (except the tortillas) and simmer on medium high for 15 minutes or until the liquids are almost evaporated.

Place a little of the mixture in the center of a tortilla and garnish with lettuce, tomato, avocado, cheese and yogurt to taste, then roll and eat.

MY CHILD CAN...

- Garnish his tortilla.

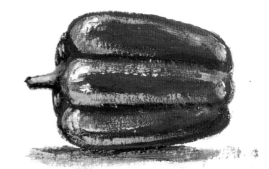

TIPS

- Double the recipe and freeze the extra meat mixture.
- To make the tortillas more savory, reheat them for 10 seconds in a large skillet on medium; flip and do other side. Or place them between damp paper towels and microwave 30 seconds.

VARIATION

- Serve the meat mixture in pita halves.

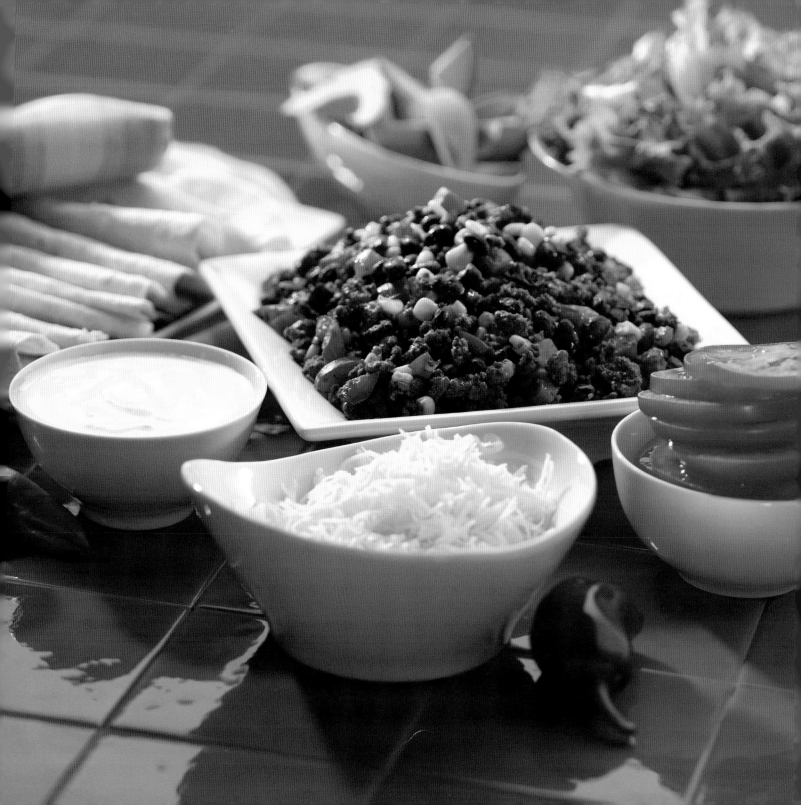

Veal

Rigatoni and Sausage Casserole

Here is a "2 in 1" recipe: a meal for dinner and another to freeze later.

340 g	(3/4 lb)	veal sausage
500 g	(1 lb)	rigatoni
10 ml	(2 tsp)	oil
1		onion, diced
2		garlic cloves, chopped
150 g	(5 oz)	chopped frozen spinach (1/2 box)
1 can	(796 ml/28 oz)	diced tomatoes
1 pinch		dried pepper flakes
1 can	(160 ml/5 oz)	evaporated milk
200 ml	(3/4 cup)	mozzarella, grated

Preheat oven to 200°C (400°F). Remove the sausage filling (throw out the casings) and crumble. Set aside.

In a large pot of boiling water, cook the rigatoni al dente. Drain and reserve.

Meanwhile, in a large skillet, heat the oil on medium and fry the onion, garlic, spinach and sausage meat just until the onion is golden and the spinach is defrosted.

Stir in the tomatoes, cooked rigatoni, pepper flakes and evaporated milk. Transfer it all to an ovenproof dish. Sprinkle with mozzarella.

Bake for 30 minutes or until the top is golden. Serve with a green salad.

MY CHILD CAN...

- Remove the sausage filling.
- Grate the cheese.

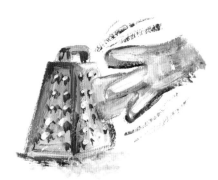

VARIATIONS

- Divide this recipe between two ovenproof casserole dishes, one for dinner and the other to freeze. Omit the mozzarella on the casserole to be frozen, cover with plastic wrap and freeze. When heating the casserole, remove the plastic wrap and replace with aluminum foil and cook without defrosting, approximately 1 hour 30 minutes. Remove the aluminum foil, sprinkle with mozzarella and place under the broiler until melted.

- To clean your grater, rinse under cold water, which will harden the cheese (hot water melts the cheese and gums up the holes of the grater!).

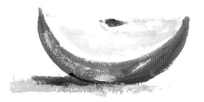

Apple Veal Cutlets

The tarragon flavored sauce highlights the delicate meat of veal and compliments the acidity of the apple.

Preparation: 10 min Cooking time: 20 min Servings: 6

10 ml	(2 tsp)	oil
6		veal cutlets (700g / 1 ½ lb total)
1		large onion, thinly sliced
2		apples, peeled and thinly sliced
250 ml	(1 cup)	chicken stock or apple juice
15 ml	(1 Tbsp)	Dijon whole grain mustard
2 ml	(1/2 tsp)	dried tarragon
		salt and pepper
45 ml	(3 Tbsp)	plain yogurt
5 ml	(1 tsp)	corn starch

In a large skillet, heat 5 ml (1 tsp) oil and sear the veal cutlets 2-3 minutes each side or until browned. Keep warm.

Add the remaining oil to the skillet and sauté the onion 5 minutes or until soft. Add the apple slices, stock, mustard and tarragon, scraping the bottom of the pan to incorporate the veal drippings. Simmer 5 minutes or until the apples are tender. Salt and pepper to taste.

Mix the yogurt and corn starch. Stir into the contents of the pan and cook 1 minute. Add the veal cutlets along with any juices remaining in the platter. Reheat all.

Serve the cutlets with rice and Carrot Ribbons (pg 72).

MY CHILD CAN...

- Peel and slice the apples under adult supervision.
- Mix the yogurt and corn starch.

TIPS

- The corn starch prevents the yogurt from curdling when heated.
- For easy removal of the apple core from a halved apple, use a melon baller. It is faster and easier than with a knife.

VARIATIONS

- Add some mushrooms and replace 125 ml (1/2 cup) of stock with white wine.
- Replace the onion with a pear.

Hunter Veal Stew

The culinary term "hunter" originated with the combination of mushrooms, tomatoes and onions.

15 ml	(3 tsp)	oil
570 g	(1 1/4 lb)	veal, cubed and floured
1		large onion, diced
1		garlic clove, chopped
1 can	(540 ml/19 oz)	diced tomatoes
1 can	(284 ml/10 oz)	sliced mushrooms, drained
15 ml	(1 Tbsp)	Dijon whole grain mustard
5 ml	(1 tsp)	Herbes de Provence
250 ml	(1 cup)	chicken stock
		salt and pepper
30 ml	(2 Tbsp)	35% cream

In a large skillet, heat 5 ml (1 tsp) oil and sear half the cubed veal until it is browned. Set aside. Add 5 ml (1 tsp) oil and sear the remaining cubes. Set aside.

Heat the remaining oil and sauté the onion and garlic until golden. Add the tomatoes and mushrooms, and cook a few minutes and stir, scraping the bottom of the pan to deglaze it. Stir in the mustard, Herbes de Provence and the chicken stock. Place the meat in the pan. Salt and pepper to taste.

Cover and let simmer 30 minutes, stirring occasionally. When cooked, stir in the cream.

Meanwhile, cook the egg noodles and broccoli.

MY CHILD CAN...
- Flour the cubed veal.

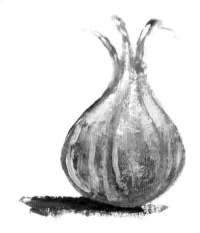

VARIATION
- You can use fresh mushrooms and replace 125 ml (1/2 cup) of stock with white wine.

Veal Burgers and Mushrooms

The secret of these juicy and savory burgers is the addition of fresh mushrooms.

Preparation: 10 min Cooking time: 15 min Servings: 8   **Can be frozen**

1 pkg	(227 g/8 oz)	fresh mushrooms
10 ml	(2 tsp)	oil
		salt
1		small onion
2		bread slices, torn up, without crusts
15 ml	(1 Tbsp)	whole grain Dijon mustard
5 ml	(1 tsp)	Herbes de Provence
500 g	(1 lb)	lean ground veal
		salt and pepper
8		hamburger buns
GARNISH		lettuce and tomato

- In a food processor, fine chop the mushrooms.

- In a non-stick pan, heat 5 ml (1 tsp) oil and sauté the mushrooms. Salt lightly.

- Again, in the food processor, fine chop the onion. Add the onion to the mushrooms and continue cooking until the liquid has evaporated.

- Put the onion mushroom mixture in a bowl, stir in the bread crumbs, mustard, Herbes de Provence and veal. Salt and pepper to taste. Form into 8 hamburger patties with your hands.

- In the same pan, add the remaining oil and heat on medium and sear the veal patties 5 minutes each side or until the meat has lost its pink color.

- Put the veal patties in the buns and garnish with lettuce and tomatoes.

MY CHILD CAN...

- Help form the veal patties.

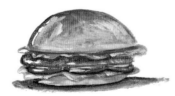

TIPS

- Double this recipe and freeze the raw patties for future use.
- Form all the patties (round or rectangular) of the same thickness: they cook more uniformly.
- Coat your hands with water or oil to avoid the meat sticking to your fingers.

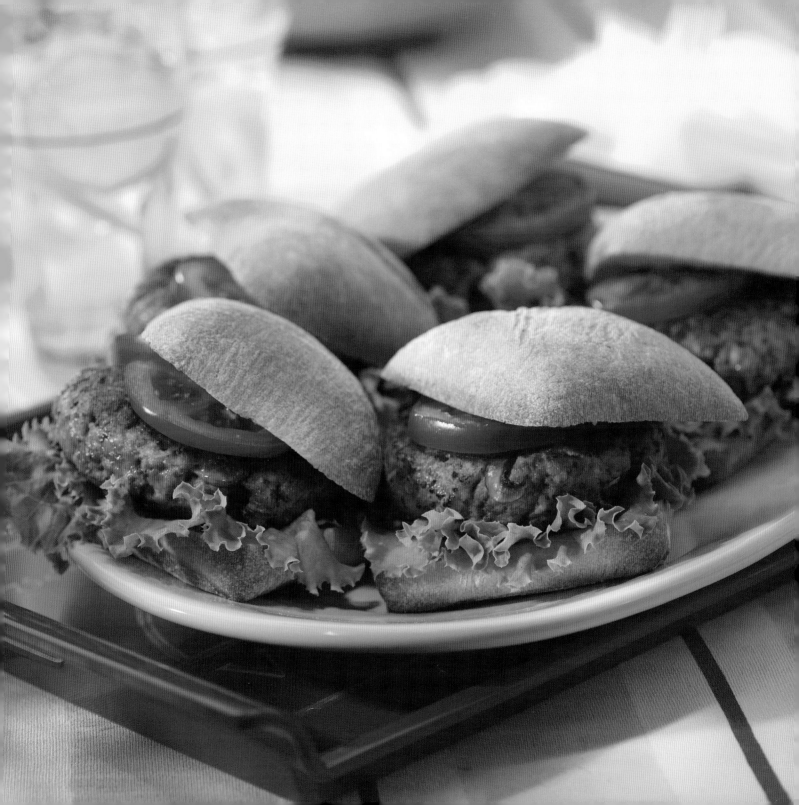

Pork

Pear and Ginger Pork Cutlets

For a different flavor, replace the pears with mango or fresh peach slices.

30 ml	(2 Tbsp)	orange juice
30 ml	(2 Tbsp)	soy sauce
15 ml	(1 Tbsp)	brown sugar
5 ml	(1 tsp)	ground ginger
5 ml	(1 tsp)	curry
1 ml	(1/4 tsp)	ground pepper
10 ml	(2 tsp)	oil
6		boned pork cutlets 700 g/1 ½ lb total
1 can	(398 ml/14 oz)	drained sliced pears
30 ml	(2 Tbsp)	chopped fresh parsley

In a small bowl, mix orange juice, soy sauce, brown sugar, ginger, curry and pepper until the sugar is dissolved. Reserve.

In a non-stick pan, heat the oil on medium. Sear the cutlets 3 minutes each side. Remove the cutlets from the pan and keep warm.

Pour the orange juice mixture in the pan and simmer 2-3 minutes or until the sauce is reduced. Stir in the pears to heat.

Serve the cutlets with the sauce and pears. Sprinkle with parsley. Delicious with Grilled Vegetables (pg 72).

MY CHILD CAN...

- Mix the sauce ingredients.

TIP

- Prepare the orange juice mixture the day before and for a more pronounced flavor, marinate the cutlets in the refrigerator overnight.

VARIATIONS

- Replace the preserved pears with 2 peeled fresh pears, cut in thick slices.
- Lovers of fresh ginger can replace the ground ginger with 15 ml (1 Tbsp) grated ginger.

Tomato Pesto Pork Cutlets

Take advantage of summer and cook these cutlets on the barbeque!

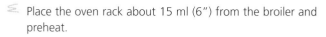

Preparation: 5 min   Baking time: 8 min   Servings: 6

6		boned pork cutlets (570 g/1 ¼ lb total)
		salt and pepper
60 ml	(4 Tbsp)	tomato pesto (commercially prepared)

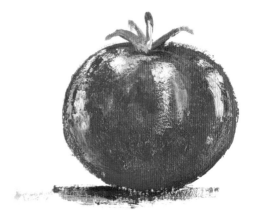

Place the oven rack about 15 ml (6") from the broiler and preheat.

Place the pork cutlets on a heavy baking sheet covered with parchment paper. Salt and pepper each side.

Broil for 4 minutes or until the meat has lost its pink color.

Remove from the oven, turn the cutlets and brush with pesto. Continue broiling about 4 minutes or until the cutlets are cooked.

Serve with Parmesan Polenta (pg 147) and Carrot Ribbons (pg 72).

MY CHILD CAN...

- Salt and pepper the cutlets.

TIP

- To freeze homemade or commercial pesto, use a plastic egg carton: fill the cavities, close the double top and freeze. Use only the quantity needed.

VARIATION

- Replace the pork with 500 g (1 lb) chicken or turkey fillets.

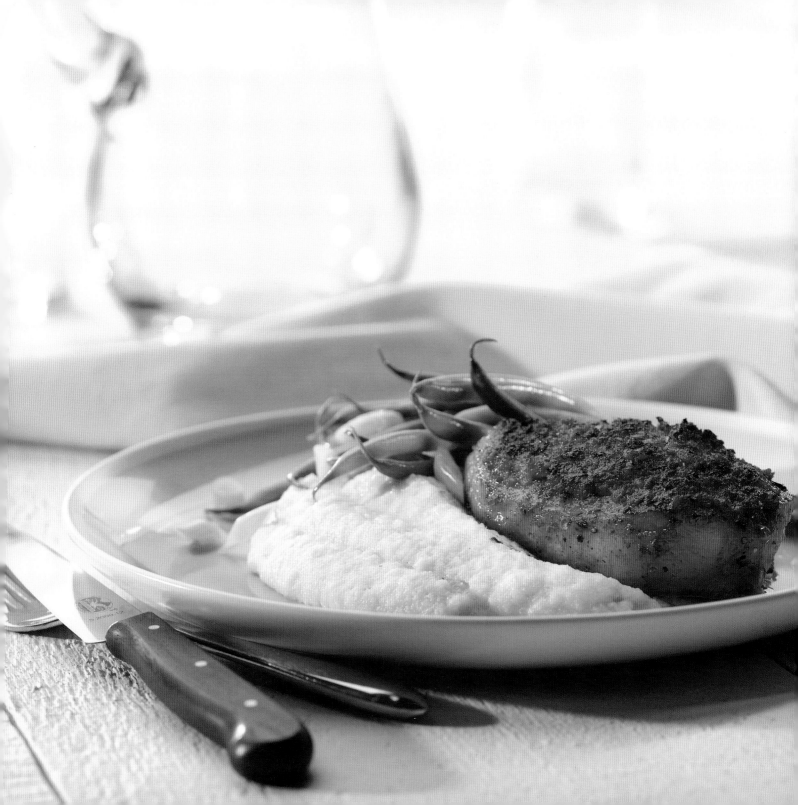

Maple Pork Tenderloin

Pork tenderloin is better served when the center is still pink.
Contrary to what one may think, it is a very lean cut.

Preparation: 10 min   Roasting time: 30 min   Servings: 6

45 ml	(3 Tbsp)	flour
5 ml	(1 tsp)	dry mustard
5 ml	(1 tsp)	sausage meat
2		pork tenderloins (700 g/1 ½ lb total)
10 ml	(2 tsp)	oil
375 ml	(1 1/2 cup)	beef stock
75 ml	(1/3 cup)	maple syrup
2		garlic cloves, finely chopped

Preheat the oven to 200°C (400°F). In a sealed plastic bag, mix the flour, mustard and sausage meat. Place the tenderloin in the bag, close, and shake well to coat with the dry mixture.

In a skillet, heat the oil on high and sear the tenderloins on all sides. Place them in an ovenproof dish.

Mix the beef stock and maple syrup, and pour over the pork. Sprinkle the tenderloins with chopped garlic.

Prepare Salted Potatoes (pg 73) and put in oven. At the same time, place the tenderloins in the oven and cook, uncovered, 30 minutes or until a meat thermometer inserted in the center of the thickest loin reads 70°C (160°F).

Transfer the pork loins to a cutting board and let rest 5 minutes. Cut into medallions 2.5 cm (1") thick. Serve with the potatoes and asparagus tips.

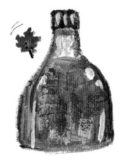

MY CHILD CAN...

- Prepare the flour mixture.
- Coat the pork loins with the flour mixture.
- Coat the potatoes with oil and salt them.

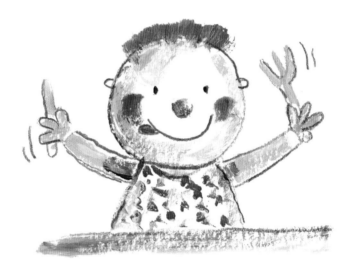

TIPS

- Test the doneness of potatoes with a fork rather than with the tip of a knife, because the knife tip will penetrate the flesh too easily and one might think that they are done when they aren't.
- Don't feel guilty if the vegetables aren't freshly gathered from the garden or bought at the market that morning.
  Profit by gaining time with frozen vegetables. On this thought, it is better to serve canned vegetables than none at all!
- You could quarter unpeeled potatoes and cook them around the pork loins.
  They will take on the flavor of the maple syrup sauce.

VARIATION

- Accompany this dish with Parmesan Polenta (pg 147).

Chicken

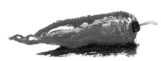

Chicken *Enchiladas*

The word *enchilada* means "seasoned with hot peppers." For a traditional more fiery version, add a finely chopped jalapeño pepper.

15 ml	(1 Tbsp)	oil
1		diced onion
1		red pepper, finely sliced
500 g	(1 lb)	skinless chicken breast cut into fine strips
300 ml	(1 1/4 cup)	commercial mild salsa
1 pkg	(125 g/4 oz)	cream cheese cut into cubes
5 ml	(1 tsp)	cumin
5 ml	(1 tsp)	chili powder
8		20 cm tortillas (8") diameter
250 ml	(1 cup)	grated mozzarella

Preheat oven to 190°C (375°F).

In a skillet, cook the onion and red pepper in the oil 5 minutes or until tender. Add the chicken and cook 5 minutes or until it has lost its pink color.

Stir in 50 ml (1/2 cup) salsa, cream cheese, cumin and chili powder. Mix well and cook just until the cheese has melted.

Place about 75 ml (1/3 cup) of the mixture in the center of each tortilla. Roll. With the fold on bottom, place in an ovenproof 23 x 33 cm (9" x 13") pan.

Cover with remaining salsa and sprinkle with the mozzarella. Bake 10 minutes in the oven or until the cheese is melted.

Serve with a carrot salad.

MY CHILD CAN...

- Cut the cheese in cubes.
- Place the filling in the center of each tortilla and roll them.

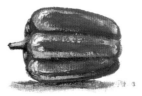

VARIATION

- You can serve this same recipe as burritos: place the filling in the center of the tortilla; fold the bottom of the tortilla on the filling and then fold the other sides toward the center. And there you are, ready to eat with your fingers!

Chinese Chicken

Inspired by Australian author Donna Hay, this flavorful recipe, fast and easy to make, adds a touch of the exotic to daily menus.

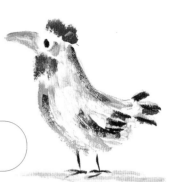

Preparation: 10 min Cooking time: 15 min Servings: 6

125 ml	(1/2 cup)	white wine or mirin
50 ml	(1/4 cup)	soy sauce
4		green onions, sliced into 1 cm (1/2") pieces
15 ml	(1 Tbsp)	fresh ginger, slivered
15 ml	(1 Tbsp)	brown sugar
10 ml	(2 tsp)	sesame oil
		red pepper flakes
500 g	(1 lb)	chicken breast, skinless

In a large non-stick skillet, mix the wine, soy sauce, green onions, ginger, brown sugar, oil and red pepper flakes. Bring to the boil.

Slice the chicken horizontally in the direction of the grain to obtain two slices of about 1 cm (1/2") thick.

Place the chicken in the skillet, forming one layer, and cook 5 minutes on medium. Turn each piece and cook 5 minutes more or until they are well cooked. Remove the chicken and keep warm.

Bring to the boil and reduce the sauce for about 3 minutes or until it is slightly sticky. Add the chicken to the pan and coat well in the sauce.

Serve with steamed rice and sliced snow peas or baby bok choy.

MY CHILD CAN...

- Peel the ginger root by scraping it with the back of a spoon.
- Cut the green onions under adult supervision.

TIP

- Begin the preparations by cooking the rice. To partly make ahead, prepare the sauce the day before and refrigerate.

VARIATIONS

- Mirin is a product with a base of vinegar, fermented rice and corn syrup. It can be found in the Asian food aisle. It can be replaced with a sweet white wine or sherry.
- Try this recipe with salmon or tuna steak or even tofu cut into approximately 1 cm (1/2") slices. Cooking time will be about the same.

Chicken *Cacciatore*

Reheated the next day and served with a variation of Grilled Polenta (variation on pg 147), this dish tastes even better...if you have any leftovers!

30 ml	(2 Tbsp)	oil
6		chicken legs, skinless
		salt and pepper
1 can	(425 ml/15 oz)	ratatouille (homemade, see pg 67)
1 can	(540 ml/19 oz)	diced tomatoes
1		bay leaf
75 ml	(1/3 cup)	red wine or stock
45 ml	(3 Tbsp)	chopped parsley

In a large saucepan, heat the oil on medium. Sear the chicken thighs 3 minutes on each side or until they are golden. Salt and pepper to taste. Remove from pan and keep warm.

In the same pan, heat the ratatouille, tomatoes, and bay leaf with the wine. Place the chicken thighs on the ratatouille. Lower the heat, cover loosely and simmer gently 30 minutes or until the chicken is well cooked.

Serve on white rice, capelli d'angelo pasta noodles or Parmesan Polenta (pg 147). Sprinkle with fresh chopped parsley.

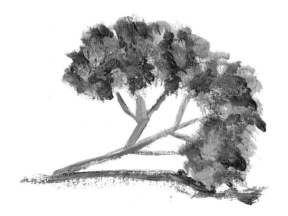

TIPS

- You can easily double this recipe and freeze in individual servings in freezer bags. It will keep up to 6 weeks. When using, defrost in the refrigerator and reheat gently in a saucepan along with a little water.

- To save time, buy skinless chicken thighs.

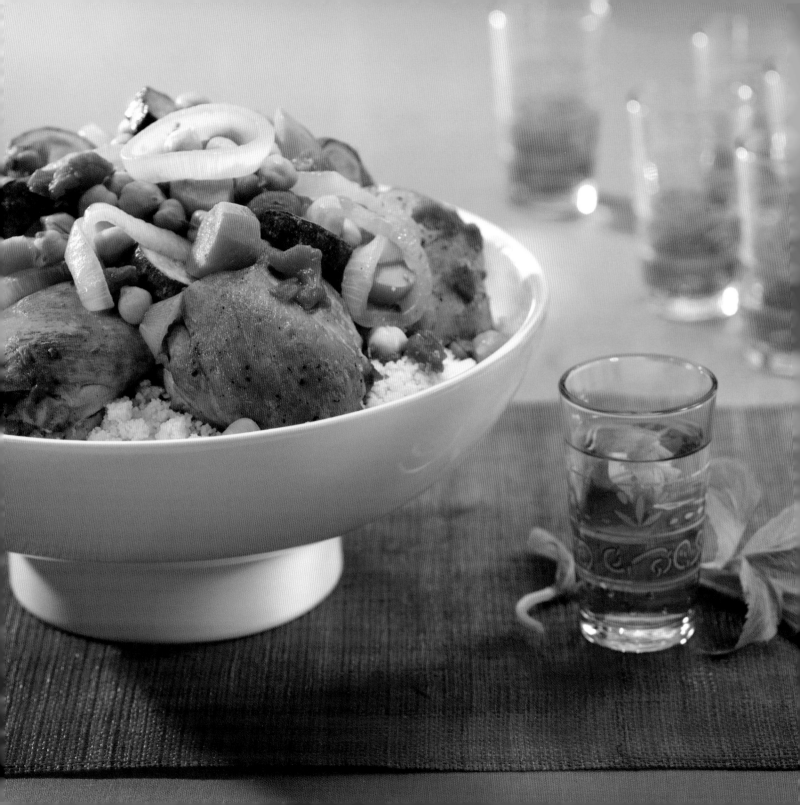

Chicken Couscous

This meal is traditionally served with hot sauce and/or harissa.

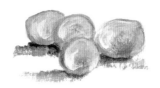

10 ml	(2 tsp)	oil
6		chicken thighs, skinless and boneless
2		large onions, finely sliced
2		carrots, sliced
2		zucchini, sliced
1 can	(540 ml/19 oz)	diced tomatoes
1 can	(540 ml/19 oz)	chick peas, rinsed and drained
500 ml	(2 cups)	chicken stock
10 ml	(2 tsp)	cumin
		cayenne to taste
		salt

In a large skillet, sear the chicken thighs in the oil on medium for 10 minutes or until golden on each side. Remove and keep warm.

In the same pan, sauté the onions on medium for 5 minutes or until golden. Add the carrots, zucchini, tomatoes, chick peas, chicken stock, cumin and cayenne.

Return the chicken thighs to the pan. Salt to taste. Cover and simmer 15 minutes or until the carrots are al dente and the chicken well done.

Serve in a nest of couscous and pour on the sauce.

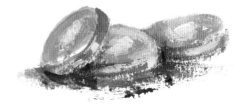

TIP

- To prepare the couscous, measure 375 ml (1 1/2 cups) of liquid (stock or salted water) per 250 ml (1 cup) dry couscous. First, boil the liquid and remove from the heat. Add the couscous, cover and let swell for approximately 5 minutes. Stir with a fork to lighten the texture and, if desired, drizzle on a little olive oil. To vary the flavor, stir in (according to your taste) fresh chopped mint, lemon zest, ground cumin or simply fresh chopped parsley.

VARIATION

- The chicken thighs can be replaced with 3 skinless chicken breasts, cut into equal large cubes.

Curry Chicken in Cream Sauce

This aromatic curry sauce owes its subtleness and creaminess to evaporated milk.

Preparation: 10 min Cooking time: 25 min Servings: 5

45 ml	(3 Tbsp)	flour
15 ml	(1 Tbsp)	curry powder
2 ml	(1/2 tsp)	salt
15 ml	(1 Tbsp)	oil
1		onion, finely sliced
2		garlic cloves, sliced
500 g	(1 lb)	chicken breasts, skinless, boneless and cubed
250 ml	(1 cup)	chicken stock
1 can	(160 ml/5 oz)	evaporated milk
15 ml	(1 Tbsp)	mango chutney or orange marmalade
15 ml	(1 Tbsp)	fresh chopped cilantro or fresh chopped parsley

In a bowl mix the flour, curry and salt. Set aside.

In a large non-stick skillet, heat the oil and fry the onions and garlic 5 minutes or until they are golden.

Meanwhile, coat the chicken pieces in the flour mixture and shake off any extra. In the skillet, add the chicken to the onions and turn until all sides are golden. Add the stock, scraping the bottom with a wooden spoon to deglaze. Stir in the milk, chutney and parsley. Bring to the boil and let simmer 10 minutes or until the sauce has thickened slightly.

Serve on basmati rice with green peas and naan, an East Indian bread similar to pita.

MY CHILD CAN...

- Mix the curry, flour and salt.
- Coat the chicken cubes in the flour mixture.

TIP

- Wash the fresh herbs only before using. Dry them well and use a well-sharpened knife to facilitate the chopping (the herbs must be chopped and not crushed with the handle of the knife).

VARIATIONS

- For a different taste, replace the chicken with lamb or veal cubes.
- For a more exotic flavor, replace the evaporated milk with coconut milk. It is available either skimmed or partially skimmed.

Chicken on Fennel

Easy and fast to prepare! Just let it cook...

1		fennel bulb, thickly sliced
3		onions, sliced
250 ml	(1 cup)	sliced mushrooms
6		chicken thighs, skinless and boneless
375 ml	(1 1/2 cup)	tomato sauce (canned or see pg 70)
75 ml	(1/3 cup)	18% cream

Preheat the oven to 180°C (350°F).

Place the sliced fennel in a shallow ovenproof pan, covering the bottom. Scatter the onions and mushrooms over the fennel. Place the chicken thighs on the vegetables. Pour on the tomato sauce and then the cream.

Bake uncovered for 50 minutes or until the chicken is cooked. Serve with green beans and egg noodles.

MY CHILD CAN...

- Cut the mushrooms with adult supervision.
- Pour the tomato sauce and cream over the chicken.

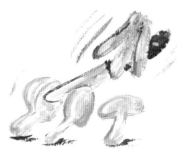

TIP

- To prepare the fennel, cut off the stems, remove the tough outer layer of the bulb, cut in two and remove the heart. The stems can be used to flavor a stock or to stuff a chicken to be roasted, and the outer layer can be chopped to be used as a garnish for soup or pasta.

VARIATION

- You can replace the chicken thighs with boneless, skinless chicken breasts, cut into large cubes.

Sesame Crusted Chicken on Salad

Tender chicken coated with crunchy sesame...this recipe will quickly become a family favorite.

Preparation: 20 min Cooking time: 10 min Servings: 6

500 g	(1 lb)	skinless chicken breast
1		egg, slightly beaten with a little water
250 ml	(1 cup)	sesame seeds
15 ml	(1 Tbsp)	oil
2		cucumbers, unpeeled
15 ml	(1 Tbsp)	rice vinegar
1 pinch		sugar
15 ml	(1 Tbsp)	minced fresh mint or 5 ml (1 tsp) dry mint
		chili flakes

- Slice the breasts horizontally in the direction of the grain to obtain two equal slices of 1 cm (1/2") thickness.
- Dip the chicken pieces in the beaten egg, then coat with sesame seeds.
- In a large skillet, heat the oil on medium. Add the chicken and cook 3-4 minutes on each side, or until they are cooked and golden.
- Using a mandolin or vegetable peeler, create thin curled slices of cucumber. Put the curls in a bowl.
- Mix the rice vinegar, sugar, mint and pepper flakes. Pour over the cucumber curls.
- Garnish dinner plates with cucumber salad placed next to the chicken.
- Serve with Chinese rice noodles or steamed rice and hoisin or plum sauce.

MY CHILD CAN...

- Coat the chicken with sesame seeds.
- Prepare the vinaigrette.

TIP

- To give the salad an Asian touch, there is nothing like the sweet and sour flavor of rice vinegar. The rice vinegar can be substituted with white wine vinegar to which a pinch of sugar is added.

VARIATIONS

- For a vegetarian version, replace the chicken with 500 g (1 lb) tofu, cut in slices of 1 cm (1/2") thickness and cook in the manner indicated.
- If time allows, marinate the chicken 30 minutes in a mix of 50 ml (1/2 cup) sake, 30 ml (2 Tbsp) soy sauce and 10 ml (2 tsp) sesame oil. Cook as indicated in the recipe.

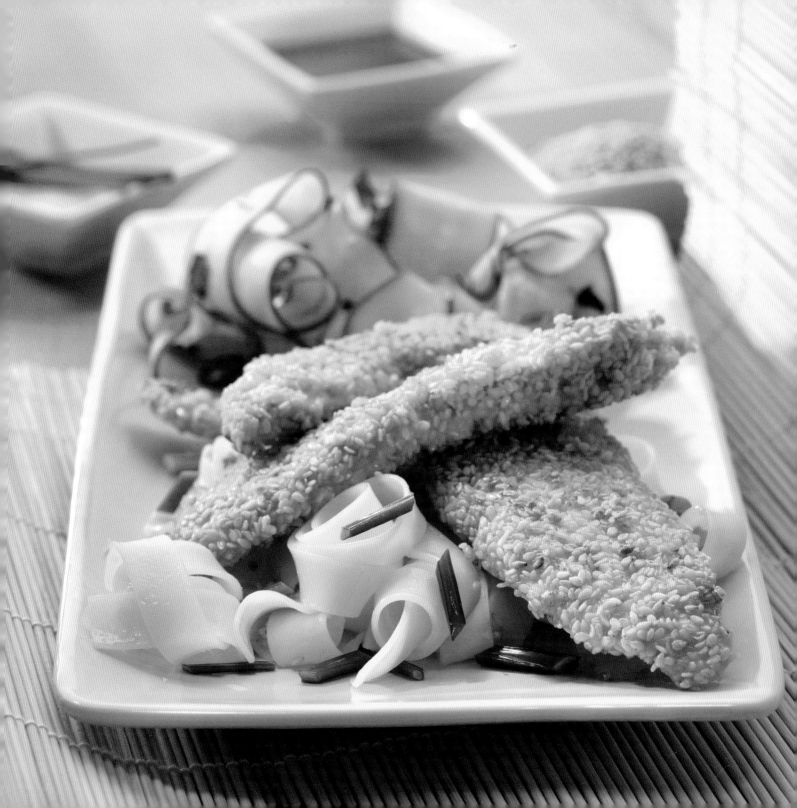

Four-Step Chicken

Only 5 minutes to prepare! And worry-free cooking that lets you whistle while you work.

Preparation: 5 min Baking time: 55 min Servings: 8   **Can be frozen**

4		skinless chicken legs with bone
		salt and pepper
		oil
8		halved Italian tomatoes
5 ml	(1 tsp)	dried basil
5 ml	(1 tsp)	dried oregano
10 ml	(2 tsp)	seasoning mix with onion (i.e. Mrs Dash) or 10 ml (2 tsp) dried chives
50 ml	(1/4 cup)	liquid (wine, stock, apple juice or water)

Preheat oven to 190°C (375°F).

Salt and pepper the chicken legs and place them in a large oiled ovenproof dish. Arrange the tomato halves around the chicken. Sprinkle seasonings over the chicken. Add the liquid.

Cover and roast for 45 minutes or until the chicken is done. Remove the cover and roast a further 10 minutes to brown the top.

Serve with Fennel Salad (pg 72) which can be prepared while the chicken is cooking.

MY CHILD CAN...
- Cut the tomatoes in half.
- Sprinkle on the seasonings and pour the liquid.

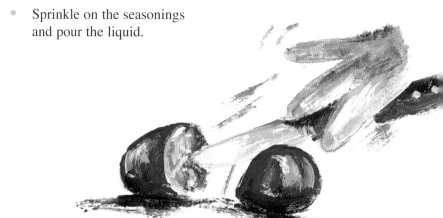

TIPS
- This dish can be prepared the night before. The next day put it in the oven.
- As a general rule, 15 ml fresh herbs can be substituted with 5 ml (1 tsp) dried herbs, a 3:1 substitution.

Mexican Roast Vegetables **and Chicken**

This savory "all in one" meal goes well with a crispy green salad.

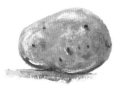

Preparation: 15 min   Baking time: 30 min   Servings: 7

60 ml	(4 Tbsp)	oil
15 ml	(1 Tbsp)	chili powder
10 ml	(2 tsp)	dried oregano
2 ml	(1/2 tsp)	salt
2		quartered onions
2		potatoes, skin on, quartered
1 pkg	(227 g/8 oz)	quartered mushrooms
1 can	(341 ml/12 oz)	kernel corn, drained or 250 ml (1 cup) frozen corn
375 ml	(1 1/2 cup)	baby carrots
30 ml	(2 Tbsp)	bread crumbs
500 g	(1 lb)	skinless chicken breast, cubed

Preheat the oven to 200°C (400°F).

In a small bowl, mix the oil, chili powder, oregano and salt. In a large bowl mix all the vegetables. Pour half the oil mixture over the vegetables and stir well to coat them. Place the vegetables in a large ovenproof dish.

Place the chicken cubes in the same large bowl. Stir the bread crumbs into the oil mixture and pour over the chicken. Stir well to coat the chicken cubes. Spread the chicken cubes on the vegetables.

Bake, uncovered in the oven, for 30 minutes or until the vegetables are roasted and the chicken done.

MY CHILD CAN...

- Cut the vegetables.
- Mix the oil and seasonings.
- Mix the vegetables and seasoned oil.

TIPS

- To prepare ahead, cube the chicken and prepare the vegetables (with the exception of the potatoes) the day before and refrigerate in separate containers.
- To prepare a variation of the Potato Frittata (pg 164) add one or two additional potatoes for the above recipe and reserve approximately 500 ml (2 cups) of the roasted vegetables.

Parmesan Chicken

The juicy chicken breasts are covered with tomato sauce and then prepared as a gratin.

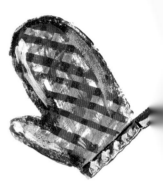

Preparation: 20 min   Baking time: 15 min   Servings: 6   **Can be frozen**

45 ml	(3 Tbsp)	bread crumbs
30 ml	(2 Tbsp)	wheat germ
10 ml	(2 tsp)	dried oregano
10 ml	(2 tsp)	dried basil
		salt and pepper
500 g	(1 lb)	skinless chicken breasts
10 ml	(2 tsp)	oil
375 ml	(1 1/2 cup)	tomato sauce (homemade see pg 70)
125 ml	(1/2 cup)	grated mozzarella
45 ml	(3 Tbsp)	grated parmesan

- Preheat the oven to 200°C (400°F).

- In a shallow baking dish, mix the bread crumbs, wheat germ, oregano, basil, salt and pepper. Set aside.

- Slice the chicken breasts horizontally in the direction of the grain to obtain two equal slices of 1 cm (1/2") thickness.

- Dip the chicken escalopes in the bread crumb mixture. In a large non-stick skillet, heat the oil and brown the escalopes approximately 2 minutes each side.

- Place in a deep ovenproof dish. Pour the tomato sauce over the escalopes. Sprinkle on the mozzarella and parmesan.

- Bake 15 minutes or until sauce bubbles and the cheese is golden.

- Serve with steamed zucchini slices and linguini drizzled with olive oil.

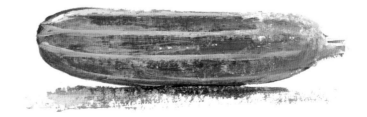

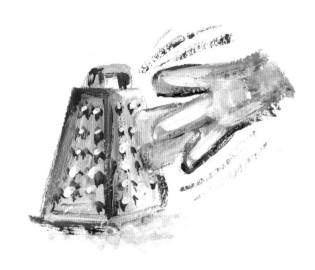

MY CHILD CAN...

- Prepare the bread crumb mixture.
- Dip the escalopes in the bread crumb mixture.
- Grate the cheese.

TIP

- To achieve the recommended 5 servings of fruit and vegetables per day, which may seem unattainable for your child, think of it as servings that are the size of a child's fist. With a fruit juice for breakfast, a fruit for snack time, and a vegetable at lunch and dinner, the goal is achieved.

VARIATIONS

- If you have a large enough skillet, leave the escalopes in the pan, pour in the tomato sauce, cover and let simmer 10 minutes. Sprinkle with cheese and cook 5 minutes longer or until the cheese is melted.
- Replace the tomato sauce with tomato slices: place the tomato slices on the chicken, then garnish with basil leaves and sprinkle with the mozzarella and parmesan cheese. Cook according to the recipe.
- For a vegetarian version, replace the chicken with 500 g (1 lb) tofu cut into 1 cm (1/2") slices and cook according to the recipe.

Turkey

Red Kidney Bean Chili

This recipe has the flavor of slow cooking but it only takes an hour.
If spicy dishes are not for you, go easy on the hot chili pepper.

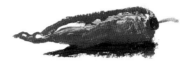

Preparation: 10 min Cooking time: 1 h Servings: 6   **Can be frozen**

15 ml	(1 Tbsp)	oil
1		diced Spanish onion
1		habanero pepper, seeded and finely chopped
2		garlic cloves, finely chopped
500 g	(1 lb)	ground turkey
15 ml	(1 Tbsp)	chili powder
15 ml	(1 Tbsp)	cumin
1		bay leaf
1		cinnamon stick
1 bottle	(341 ml/12 oz)	your favorite dark beer
1 can	(540 ml/19 oz)	kidney beans, rinsed and drained
GARNISH		fresh diced tomato, fresh chopped cilantro, and plain yogurt

In a large saucepan, brown the onions in oil for 5 minutes or until tender. Add the hot pepper and garlic and cook 3 minutes or until the pepper is tender.

Add the ground turkey and the spices, and cook until the turkey has lost its pink color.

Stir in the beer, scraping the bottom of the pot to deglaze. Add the red kidney beans. Bring to the boil, lower the heat and simmer 45 minutes, stirring occasionally. Add water to thin the consistency if necessary.

Remove the cinnamon stick and the bay leaf. Serve with the diced tomatoes, fresh cilantro and plain yogurt.

Makes 1.5 L (6 cups).

VARIATIONS

- Vegetarian version: replace the turkey with a package of vegetarian "turkey." Add only at the end of the cooking time, as it is precooked.
- Hot peppers owe their heat to the seeds and the white membrane (placenta) within the pods. For a really hot dish, use the whole chili pepper; for less heat, remove the seeds and membranes.

TIPS

- Avoid touching the face, mouth or eyes after handling the habanero pepper. You might also want to use rubber gloves while handling hot peppers.
- To moderate the heat of peppers, nothing works better than drinking milk, which contains a soothing substance called casein.

Turkey *Piccata*

This quick low-fat dish will become a family classic.

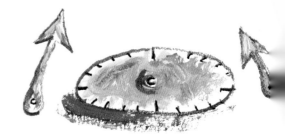

Preparation: 10 min   Cooking time: 10 min   Servings: 4

4		slices of turkey breast, 1 cm (1/2") thick (500 g/1 lb total)
45 ml	(3 Tbsp)	flour
		salt and pepper
10 ml	(2 tsp)	oil
1		chopped garlic clove
125 ml	(1/2 cup)	chicken stock
		juice of 1 lemon
15 ml	(1 Tbsp)	capers
2 ml	(1/2 tsp)	sugar
10 ml	(2 tsp)	butter
15 ml	(1 Tbsp)	fresh chopped parsley

Flour, salt and pepper the turkey slices.

In a large skillet, heat the oil on medium and sear the turkey 2-3 minutes each side. Set aside and keep warm.

In the same skillet, fry the garlic a few seconds. Add the stock, deglazing the bottom of the pan. Cook 1 minute and add the lemon juice, capers and sugar. Cook 30 seconds more and add the butter.

Pour the sauce on the turkey, sprinkle with parsley and serve with steamed broccoli and Parmesan Polenta (pg 147).

MY CHILD CAN...

- Juice the lemon.
- Flour the turkey.

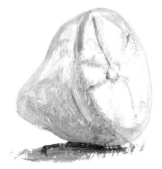

TIP

- To assure uniform cooking, be sure to maintain the same thickness of turkey; also, slice them horizontally with the grain or flatten them.

VARIATION

- This sauce would also be savory with a white fish fillet.

Mexican Macaroni

Ground turkey is inexpensive and is the leanest of the ground meats.

500 ml	(2 cups)	macaroni
1		medium onion, diced
225 g	(1/2 lb)	ground turkey
10 ml	(2 tsp)	oil
1 can	(227 ml/8 oz)	marinated bean salad or 250 ml (1 cup) cooked beans
1 can	(213 ml/7 1/2 oz)	tomato sauce
1 can	(540 ml/19 oz)	diced tomatoes
15 ml	(1 Tbsp)	chili powder
50 ml	(1/4 cup)	fresh chopped parsley

In a large saucepan of boiling water, cook the pasta until it is al dente. Drain and keep warm.

Meanwhile, cook the onion and turkey in oil until the turkey has lost its pink color and the onion is soft. Stir in the beans, tomato sauce, diced tomatoes, chili powder and the cooked macaroni. Mix well and cook a few minutes to heat all the ingredients. Stir in the fresh parsley and serve.

VARIATIONS

- For a vegetarian version, replace the turkey with a package (340 g/12 oz) of vegetarian "turkey." Add at the end of cooking as it is already cooked.
- For a fiery version, sauté a finely chopped jalapeno pepper with the onion and turkey.

Meat Loaf

This is a family favorite. As a fast accompaniment, slip some potatoes in the oven at the same time as the meat loaf.

Preparation: 10 min Baking time: 1 h Servings: 10   **Can be frozen**

2		eggs
30 ml	(2 Tbsp)	Dijon mustard
4		chopped green onions
570 g	(1 1/4 lb)	ground turkey
340 g	(3/4 lb)	ground veal
125 ml	(1/2 cup)	wheat germ
30 ml	(2 Tbsp)	chopped capers
2 ml	(1/2 tsp)	ground sage
5 ml	(1 tsp)	salt
50 ml	(1/4 cup)	cranberry sauce (canned or homemade)
		whole unpeeled potatoes

Preheat the oven to 180°C (350°F).

In a bowl mix the eggs and mustard. Stir in the green onions, turkey, veal, wheat germ, capers, sage and salt.

Spread in a 28 x 10 cm (11" x 4") loaf pan. In the center of the loaf, make a lengthwise trough and fill with the cranberry sauce.

Place the meat loaf on a baking sheet and put the potatoes around the loaf pan. Bake for 1 hour or until the potatoes are cooked and a meat thermometer reads 70°C (160°F) when inserted in the middle of the meat loaf.

Serve with remaining cranberry sauce and broccoli.

MY CHILD CAN...

- Mix the egg and Dijon mustard.
- Make the trough and fill with cranberry sauce.

TIP

- Prepare two meat loaves at the same time. Cut the second into slices and freeze individually.

VARIATION

- Replace the cranberry sauce with a sweet and sour sauce. In a saucepan, mix 1 can (398 ml/14 oz) diced tomatoes, 1 small finely chopped onion, 50 ml (1/4 cup) red wine vinegar and 5 ml (1 tsp) honey. Bring to a boil on medium. Reduce the heat and simmer, stirring for 10 minutes until it has thickened. Salt and pepper to taste. Brush the top of the meat loaf with approximately 30 ml (2 Tbsp) of the sauce before baking. Serve the remaining sauce as an accompaniment. This makes about 500 ml (2 cups) of sauce.

Asian Turkey Roll

The meat and the tortillas freeze. Why not double this recipe and have a meal on hand!

10 ml	(2 tsp)	oil
500 g	(1 lb)	ground turkey
30 ml	(2 Tbsp)	fresh chopped ginger
2		chopped garlic cloves
6		sliced green onions
45 ml	(3 Tbsp)	hoisin sauce
15 ml	(1 Tbsp)	orange juice frozen concentrate, defrosted
30 ml	(2 Tbsp)	water
6		tortillas (20 cm/8" diameter)
GARNISH		lettuce leaves, grated carrots

In a large non-stick skillet, sauté the ground turkey in 5 ml (1 tsp) oil for 10 minutes or until the turkey has lost its pink color. Strain off the fat and reserve the ground turkey.

In the same skillet, heat the remaining oil and sauté the ginger and garlic 30 seconds or until the mixture smells pungent. Add the green onions, hoisin sauce, orange juice, water and reserved turkey. Cook a few minutes to heat all the ingredients.

Serve in the warmed tortillas, garnish with lettuce and grated carrots.

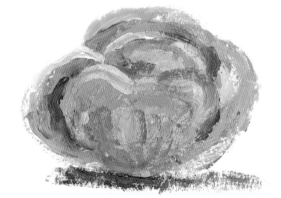

TIP
- Choose a good-sized piece of ginger with a smooth slightly shiny skin.

VARIATIONS
- Replace the lettuce with grated cabbage and the carrots with slices of red or yellow bell pepper.
- For a "spring roll" version, replace the tortillas with rehydrated 24 cm (9 ½") rice paper galette.
- For a more solid roll, use 2 rice paper galettes. Be sure that the meat mixture is not too hot before making the rolls.

Fish

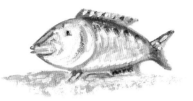

Tuna Croque-Monsieur

Light flaked tuna (yellow fin tuna) as used in this recipe contains 3 times less mercury than solid white tuna (albacore tuna).

Preparation: 10 min Baking time: 3 min Servings: 4

4		whole wheat bread
1 can	(170 g/6 oz)	light flake tuna well drained
1		green onion, finely chopped
45 ml	(3 Tbsp)	mayonnaise
45 ml	(3 Tbsp)	dill pickle finely chopped
		salt and pepper
1		sliced tomato
		a few red onion rings
125 ml	(1/2 cup)	old cheddar, grated

Preheat the broiler.

Toast the bread slices in a toaster.

In a bowl, mix the tuna with the green onion, mayonnaise and chopped dill pickle. Salt and pepper to taste. Spread the mixture on the toasted bread.

On each slice, place 2 tomato slices, a few red onion rings and sprinkle on the grated cheese.

Place under the broiler and grill just until the cheese bubbles. Serve with Fennel Salad (pg 72).

MY CHILD CAN...

- Prepare the tuna mix.
- Spread the toast with tuna mix.
- Place the tomato slices on top.
- Grate the cheese.

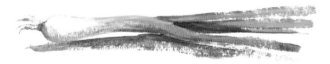

VARIATIONS

- For a brunch, use pumpernickel bread, replace the tuna with smoked salmon, garnish with red onion rings and a few chunks of cream cheese (omit the cheddar) before putting under the grill.
- Replace the mayonnaise with plain yogurt.

Asian Salmon Croquettes

This unique recipe is a source of omega 3 good fat.

Preparation: 15 min Cooking time: 10 min Servings: 6   **Can be frozen**

2 cans	(213 g/ 7 1/2 oz ea.)	drained salmon, preferably sockeye
2		bread slices, no crusts, torn into bits
1		egg, beaten
20 ml	(4 tsp)	hoisin sauce
2		green onions, finely chopped
15 ml	(1 Tbsp)	fresh ginger, finely chopped
5 ml	(1 tsp)	sesame oil
2		garlic cloves, finely chopped
		oil

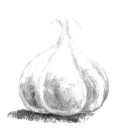

Drain the salmon and, if desired, remove the skin and the bones. (By keeping the bones, you benefit from their calcium.) Stir in the remaining ingredients. Mix well, flaking the salmon, until all is combined. Form 6 croquettes of about 2 cm (3/4") thick, pressing together well with your hands.

Cover the bottom of a skillet with a good coat of oil and heat on medium. Fry the croquettes 5 minutes each side until they are golden (turn with a large spatula, taking care not to break them).

Serve on a bed of lettuce or shredded napa cabbage with julienned carrots, rice vermicelli and the following recipe of sesame mayonnaise as an accompaniment.

Sesame Mayonnaise

Mix 30 ml (2 Tbsp) mayonnaise with 30 ml (2 Tbsp) plain yogurt, 2 ml (1/2 tsp) soy sauce, 2 ml (1/2 tsp) sesame oil and 5 ml (1 tsp) sesame seeds.

MY CHILD CAN...

- Tear up the bread slices (and eat the crusts!).
- Form the croquettes.
- Prepare the sesame mayonnaise.

TIP

- Fresh ginger will keep up to 3 weeks in the refrigerator when stored in a plastic bag or 3 months in the freezer. When needed, slice off the desired amount and store the remainder.

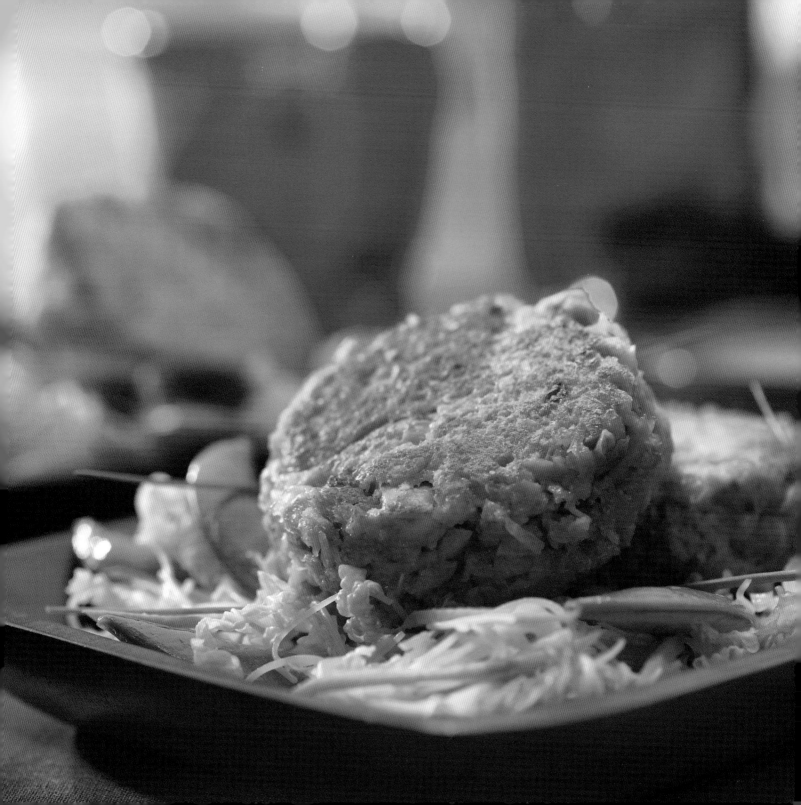

Fish Fillets with Herb Sauce

Ideal for a rushed dinner! This fish dish is prepared and cooked in the microwave in just 15 minutes.

Preparation: 10 min Cooking time: 5 min Servings: 5   **Can be frozen**

10 ml	(2 tsp)	oil
700 g	(1 1/2 lb)	fish fillets (halibut, cod or sole)
45 ml	(3 Tbsp)	soft butter
30 ml	(2 Tbsp)	fresh chopped parsley or 10 ml (2 tsp) dried parsley
30 ml	(2 Tbsp)	fresh chopped chives or 10 ml (2 tsp) dried chives
15 ml	(1 Tbsp)	lemon juice
10 ml	(2 tsp)	whole grain Dijon mustard
		salt and pepper
50 ml	(1/4 cup)	white wine or chicken stock
		lemon quarters

- In a large oiled microwave-proof dish, arrange the fish in a single layer.
- In a bowl, prepare the herb butter by mixing the butter, parsley, chives, lemon juice and Dijon mustard, forming a spread. Salt and pepper to taste. Cover the fish with this mixture. Pour on the white wine.
- Cover and microwave, on high, 5-6 minutes or until the fish is cooked.
- Drizzle on lemon juice, to your taste, and serve with brown rice, brussels sprouts and lemon quarters.

MY CHILD CAN...

- Mix the ingredients for the herb butter and spread on the fish.

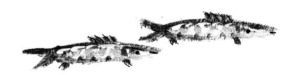

TIPS

- Know when a fish is cooked? While cooking, the flesh will lose its shiny and translucent look and will become opaque and firm when done.
- Double or triple the ingredients for the herb butter, form into nut-sized balls and store up to 3 months in the freezer.

VARIATION

- For an Asian flavor, replace the lemon juice with lime juice, the whole grain mustard with fresh ground pepper and the parsley with fresh cilantro. Add a little lemon or lime zest.

Grilled Salmon with Yogurt Sauce

This tantalizing dish with its unique flavors, is ready in less than a quarter of an hour.

200 ml	(3/4 cup)	plain yogurt
45 ml	(3 Tbsp)	fresh parsley, chopped
30 ml	(2 Tbsp)	lemon juice
30 ml	(2 Tbsp)	oil
5 ml	(1 tsp)	cumin
2		garlic cloves, finely chopped
		salt and pepper
500 g	(1 lb)	fresh salmon fillets
2		romaine hearts (in leaves)
		lemon quarters

In a bowl, mix the yogurt, parsley, lemon juice, 10 ml (2 tsp) oil, cumin and the garlic. Salt and pepper to taste. Set aside.

Brush the salmon fillets with 10 ml (2 tsp) oil. Salt and pepper to taste.

Heat the remaining oil on medium in a non-stick skillet. Place the salmon fillets, skin side down, in the pan, then cover and cook 5-7 minutes or until the flesh is almost opaque throughout.

Arrange on a bed of romaine lettuce with lemon quarters, garnish with the yogurt sauce and serve. Accompany with Grilled Vegetables (pg 72).

MY CHILD CAN...

- Prepare the yogurt sauce.
- Arrange lettuce on the plates.

TIPS

- By keeping the skin of the salmon on the fillets, you protect the delicate flesh and assure the fillet remains in one piece. Once the fish is cooked, the skin is easily removed.
- Double the ingredients for the yogurt sauce: it will also serve as a salad dressing.

VARIATIONS

- Replace the salmon fillets with fresh tuna steaks and cook in the same manner.
- The next day, serve the leftover salmon steaks as a salad with romaine lettuce, some cherry tomatoes and the yogurt sauce.

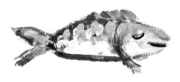

Catalan Fish

Don't be awed by the title. This is a fast and easy recipe requiring only very fresh fish.

Preparation: 10 min   Baking time: 10 min   Servings: 5   **Can be frozen**

20 ml	(4 tsp)	oil
700 g	(1 1/2 lb)	fish fillets (halibut, cod or sole)
1		small onion, finely chopped
1		garlic clove, finely chopped
50 ml	(1/4 cup)	white wine or chicken stock
1 can	(540 ml/19 oz)	diced tomatoes
8		chopped black olives
2 ml	(1/2 tsp)	dried oregano
		salt and pepper

Preheat oven to 260°C (500°F).

Oil a large ovenproof dish with 10 ml (2 tsp) oil and place the fillets in it in a single layer.

In a large skillet, heat the remaining oil on medium and fry the onions 5 minutes or until golden. Add the garlic and wine and simmer 1 minute. Stir in the tomatoes, olives and oregano. Salt and pepper to taste.

Cover the fish with this mixture. Bake 10 minutes or until the fish is cooked.

Serve immediately with brown rice or Herb and Lemon Orzo (pg 139) and some green beans.

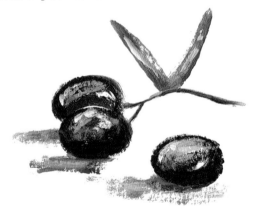

TIP
- The bran and germ of brown rice gives it an agreeable nutty flavor and carries a good dose of vitamins, minerals and fiber. To avoid it going rancid, store in the refrigerator.

VARIATION
- Replace the canned tomatoes with fresh diced Roma or plum tomatoes.

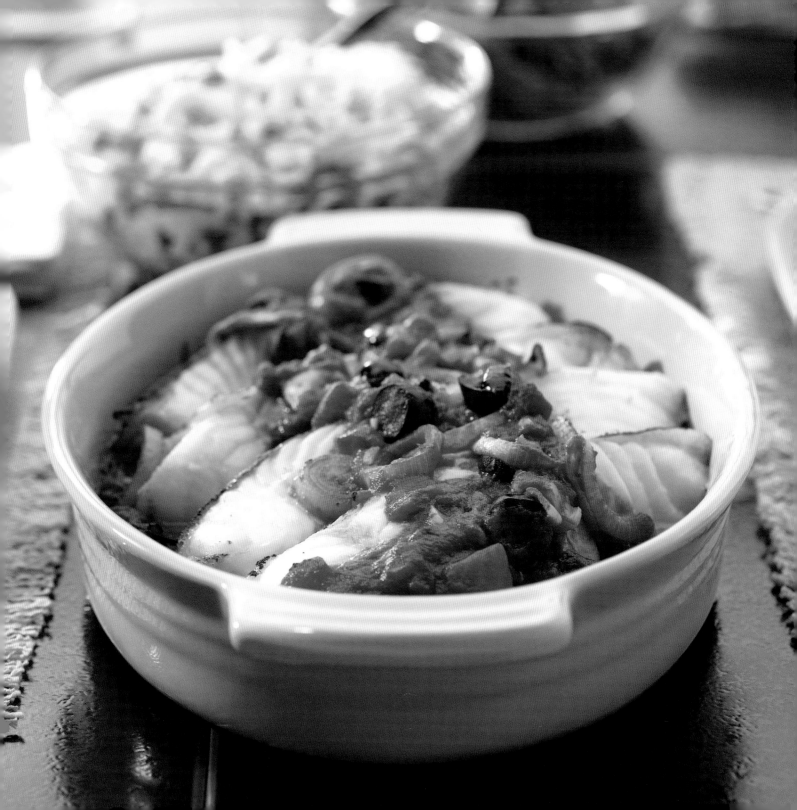

Pasta and pizzas

Herb and Lemon Orzo

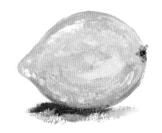

Orzo is a pasta that resembles rice grains.
The name is Italian meaning "bird's tongue."

375 ml	(1 1/2 cup)	orzo
30 ml	(2 Tbsp)	fresh chopped parsley
30 ml	(2 Tbsp)	fresh chopped chives
10 ml	(2 tsp)	oil
5 ml	(1 tsp)	lemon zest
		salt and pepper

In a large pot of boiling salted water, cook the orzo 8 minutes or until al dente. Drain and place in a serving bowl. Stir in the remaining ingredients. Salt and pepper to taste.

Serve as an accompaniment to Tomato Pesto Pork Cutlets (pg 106) or Grilled Salmon with Yogurt Sauce (pg 135).

MY CHILD CAN...

- Scissor-cut the chives.

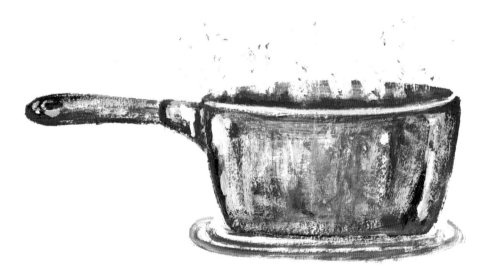

VARIATION

- To prepare as a salad dish, add 500 ml (2 cups) bite-sized cooked chicken pieces or a can of light tuna, well drained; also add 375 ml (1 1/2 cups) cooked beans cut in 2 cm (3/4") pieces, some black olives and halved cherry tomatoes.

Pan Fusilli

Whole wheat pasta contains 3 times the fiber of regular pasta, satisfies your hunger and is the far healthier choice.

Preparation: 10 min Cooking time: 20 min Servings: 6   Can be frozen

10 ml	(2 tsp)	oil
400 g	(14 oz)	ground beef
1		small sliced leek
1		chopped garlic clove
500 ml	(2 cups)	whole wheat fusilli, penne or macaroni
1		zucchini, sliced
125 ml	(1/2 cup)	sliced celery
1 boîte	(796 ml/28 oz)	diced tomatoes
15 ml	(1 Tbsp)	Worcestershire sauce
5 ml	(1 tsp)	Herbes de Provence
250 ml	(1 cup)	water
		salt and pepper

In a large skillet, heat the oil on medium and cook the ground beef. Cook 3 minutes or until it is lightly browned.

Add the leek, garlic and pasta and cook 2 minutes, stirring well to coat all with oil.

Add the zucchini, celery, tomatoes, Worcestershire sauce, Herbes de Provence and water. Salt and pepper to taste. Bring to the boil, lower the heat, cover and simmer 15 minutes or until the pasta is cooked. Stir from time to time, adding a little water if needed.

MY CHILD CAN...

- Slice the zucchini in rounds under adult supervision.

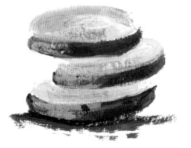

VARIATIONS

- For a vegetarian version, replace the ground beef with a package of Veggie Round Ground. Add at the end of cooking as it is already cooked.

- For a creamier version, stir in 200 ml (3/4 cup) milk at the end of cooking and reheat before serving.

- Replace the zucchini slices with 375 ml (1 1/2 cups) green beans cut in 4 cm (1 1/2") long pieces.

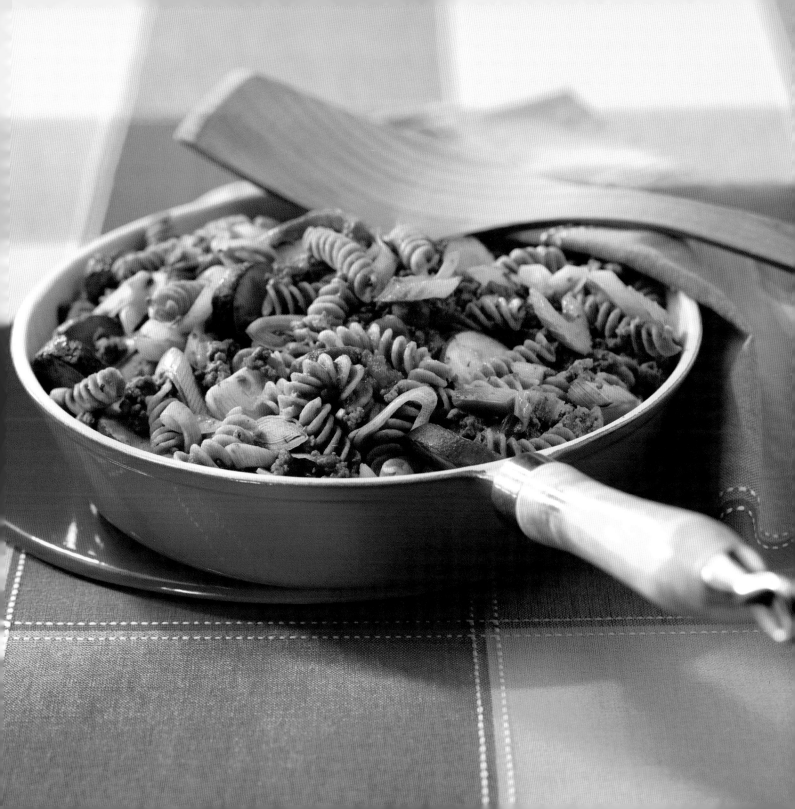

Pizza Dough

No store bought product can beat this homemade dough! For a stuffed crust, restaurant-quality pizza, incorporate cheese strips into the crust as you are forming it.

Preparation: 10 min (Resting time 10 min) Servings: 4 (500 g/1 lb)   **Can be frozen**

250 ml	(1 cup)	flour
250 ml	(1 cup)	whole wheat flour
1 envelope		yeast or quick rise instant yeast
5 ml	(1 tsp)	salt
2 ml	(1/2 tsp)	sugar
200 ml	(3/4 cup)	water
5 ml	(1 tsp)	oil

In a food processor, mix the flours, yeast, salt and sugar. Set aside.

Heat the water and oil in the microwave 1 minute on high (the temperature of the water should reach 52-55°C / 125-130°F).

While running the food processor, add the water and oil and blend until a dough ball is formed. Continue running for 1 minute to knead the dough.

Transfer the dough to a floured surface, cover with plastic wrap and let rest 10 minutes. Roll out and form your pizza.

This makes a large pizza or 2 individual pizzas or 2 calzones.

MY CHILD CAN...

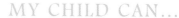

- Press the food processor buttons.
- Stir in the liquid.
- Form the pizza dough.

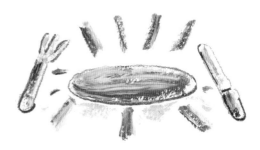

TIPS

- Remember not to overheat the water in the microwave. Water which is too hot kills the action of the yeast, whereas water which is too cold will not activate the yeast.

- Prepare the dough the night before and refrigerate in a sealed plastic bag. Before using, let it rest at room temperature for 15 minutes. For topping ideas, see next page.

- Prepare several dough batches and freeze them in individual sealed plastic bags. You now have a ready supply on hand for a quick pizza.

Pizza Party!

Delivery guaranteed in less than 30 minutes!

| 500 g | (1 lb) | fresh pizza dough (commercial or see facing page) |

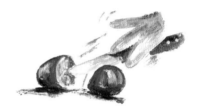

- Preheat the oven to 230°C (450°F).
- Generously sprinkle corn meal on a baking sheet forming a 33 cm (13") diameter or make a parchment paper circle.
- Roll the dough into a 30 cm (12") circle and place it on the prepared baking sheet. Form a crust from the dough and oil lightly.
- Top with desired garnishes and top this with grated cheese.
- Bake for 10-12 minutes or until the cheese is bubbling.
- Makes one 30 cm (12") pizza or two 15 cm (6") pizzas.

GARNISHING IDEAS

- **Pesto**
  Garnish: 45 ml (3 Tbsp) basil pesto and 4 sliced roma tomatoes

  Cheese: 250 ml (1 cup) grated fontina or havarti

- **Provençal**
  Garnish: 250 ml (1 cup) canned ratatouille (or see p. 67) and 50 ml (1/4 cup) sliced black olives

  Cheese: 250 ml (1 cup) grated provolone and 50 ml (1/4 cup) grated parmesan

- **Margharita**
  Garnish: 50 ml (1/4 cup) tomato sauce and approximately one dozen fresh whole basil leaves

  Cheese: 250 ml (1 cup) grated mozzarella

- **Artichoke**
  Garnish: 50 ml (1/4 cup) tomato sauce, one bottle marinated baby artichokes, drained and quartered, and 30 ml (2 Tbsp) grilled pine nuts

  Cheese: 125 ml (1/2 cup) parmesan and 125 ml (1/2 cup) grated asiago (or old cheddar)

- **Pepperoni–Cheese**
  Garnish: 50 ml (1/4 cup) tomato sauce and one dozen slices vegetarian pepperoni

  Cheese: 250 ml (1 cup) grated mozzarella

- **Chicken–Apple**
  Garnish: 15 ml (1 Tbsp) olive oil (to brush the dough), 90 g (3 oz) cooked chicken, ½ apple sliced and some toasted walnuts

  Cheese: 250 ml (1 cup) grated gruyère

- **Pear–Blue Cheese**
  Garnish: 15 ml (1 Tbsp) olive oil (to brush the dough), ½ pear sliced and 30 ml (2 Tbsp) toasted pine nuts

  Cheese: 90 g (3 oz) crumbled blue cheese and 125 ml (1/2 cup) grated mozzarella

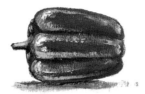

Roasted Peppers and Chicken Pasta

For a vegetarian meal, replace the chicken with 75 ml (1/3 cup) toasted pine nuts and 125 ml (1/2 cup) crumbled feta.

144

Preparation: 10 min Cooking time: 10 min Servings: 6

1 pkg	(375 g)	long pasta (capelli d'angelo, linguine)
125 ml	(1/2 cup)	basil pesto
15 ml	(1 Tbsp)	oil
2		garlic cloves, finely sliced
500 ml	(2 cups)	cooked chicken strips
125 ml	(1/2 cup)	black olives, pitted and halved
1 pot	(170 ml/6 oz)	roasted red peppers, drained and sliced
		salt and pepper
		grated parmesan

In a large pot of salted boiling water, cook the pasta until it is al dente. Reserve 250 ml (1 cup) of the cooking water, drain the pasta and keep warm.

Dilute the pesto in the reserved cooking water. Set aside.

Meanwhile, in a large skillet, heat the oil on medium and cook the garlic 30 seconds or until it smells pungent. Stir in the chicken and olives and cook 3 minutes while stirring just until all is well heated.

Add the pasta, peppers and diluted pesto to the contents in the skillet and mix well.

Salt and pepper to taste.

Sprinkle with parmesan and serve immediately, accompanied by a green salad.

MY CHILD CAN...

- Mix the pesto and cooking water.
- Slice the pitted olives and cut them in two.

TIP

- To pit the olives easily, give them a good bang with the flat of the blade of a large knife. The olive will split in two, exposing the pit.

VARIATION

- Replace the chicken with canned flaked tuna.

Presto Tuna and Tomato Pasta
— *Spaghetti al tonno e pomodoro*

Leftovers (if there are any) slip easily into the lunch box for next day.

1 pkg	(375 g)	long pasta (linguine, capelli d'angelo, spaghettini)
2 cans	(170 g/ 6 oz ea.)	flaked light tuna, drained
1 container	(380 ml)	bruschetta (commercial)
30 ml	(2 Tbsp)	35% cream
		grated parmesan

In a large pot of salted boiling water, cook the pasta until al dente. Drain and put back in the cooking pot.

Stir in the tuna, bruschetta and cream. Mix well, reheat and serve with parmesan.

MY CHILD CAN...

- Test the doneness of the pasta.

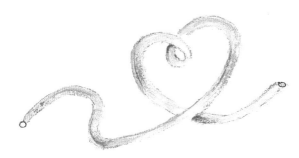

TIP

- One serving of long dried pasta is a little larger in diameter than a 25-cent piece. For short pasta, calculate approximately 200 ml (3/4 cup) per serving.

VARIATION

- Replace the tuna with the same quantity of canned salmon.

Creamy Pesto Sauce Pasta

To accelerate the preparation of dinner, start to heat the cooking water for the pasta before preparing the sauce.

Preparation: 5 min Cooking time: 10 min Servings: 6   **Vegetarian**

1 pkg	(450 g)	long pasta (linguine, fettuccini)
750 ml	(3 cups)	milk
60 ml	(4 Tbsp)	flour
1 pkg	(125 g/4 oz)	cream cheese, cut in cubes
45 ml	(3 Tbsp)	basil pesto
		salt and pepper
125 ml	(1/2 cup)	toasted pine nuts
		grated parmesan

In a large pot of salted boiling water, cook the pasta until al dente. Drain and keep warm.

Meanwhile, in a saucepan, mix the milk and flour with a whisk. Heat on medium high while stirring constantly until the sauce simmers and thickens.

Add the cheese cubes and stir until they have melted.

Stir in the pesto. Pour the sauce over reserved pasta and mix well. Salt and pepper to taste. Garnish with pine nuts and grated parmesan and serve.

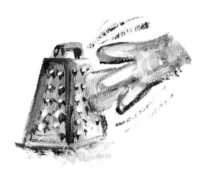

TIPS
- When reheating this pasta, add a small amount of milk, making the sauce a little creamier.
- When nuts are oven toasted, their flavor is enhanced. Spread them on a baking sheet and place in a 180°C (350°F) oven for 5-8 minutes. Or pan roast them in a frying pan on medium heat, while stirring often, for 3-4 minutes. You can also place the nuts on a plate and microwave them 4-5 minute on high. In any case, the nuts are ready when browned and take on a nutty aroma.

VARIATIONS
- For a different flavor, replace the basil pesto with tomato pesto.
- Replace half the cubed cream cheese with grated fontina, a mild nut flavored cheese which melts well.
- Serve this pasta with spiced veal sausage, chorizo sausage or a few bacon slices or prosciutto cooked separately.

Parmesan Polenta

Here is the perfect accompaniment for roast pork or lamb, or grilled sausages.

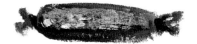

500 ml	(2 cups)	water
625 ml	(2 1/2 cups)	chicken stock
2 ml	(1/2 tsp)	salt
10 ml	(2 tsp)	butter
250 ml	(1 cup)	instant polenta (or precooked corn meal)
125 ml	(1/2 cup)	grated parmesan
		pepper

In a large saucepan, bring the water and stock to the boil. Add the salt and butter and lower the heat to medium.

Add the polenta in a stream, while stirring constantly, for 5 minutes or until the polenta detaches from the sides of the saucepan.

Remove from heat and stir in the parmesan. Pepper to taste.

Serve immediately accompanied by Chicken Cacciatore (pg 113) or Turkey Piccata (pg 126).

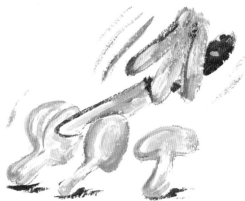

VARIATIONS

- Garnish the polenta with 500 ml (2 cups) sliced mushrooms (button, porcini, etc.) sautéed in a little oil seasoned with 2 ml (1/2 tsp) thyme and 5 ml (1 tsp) balsamic vinegar.

- Replace the parmesan with the same amount of grated fontina.

- Grill the polenta. To do this, pour the hot polenta into a pyrex dish which has been rinsed in cold water and not wiped. Once the polenta is solid, turn it out and cut into slices. Grill the sliced polenta in the oven or fry in an oiled pan. Garnish with tomato sauce, walnuts or gorgonzola, and serve.

Deluxe Tomato Ravioli

This tomato sauce also goes well with linguine, garnished with some large plump shrimp.

Preparation: 5 min Cooking time: 25 min Servings: 7

**Vegetarian
Can be frozen**

2 pkg	(454 g ea.)	frozen cheese ravioli or tortellini
500 ml	(2 cups)	tomato sauce (commercial or see pg 70)
45 ml	(3 Tbsp)	sundried tomato pesto
5 ml	(1 tsp)	sugar
125 ml	(1/2 cup)	18% cream
		pepper
		grated parmesan

- In a large pot of salted boiling water, cook the ravioli until al dente. Drain and keep warm.

- In the same pot, heat the tomato sauce with the pesto and sugar. Stir in the cream and cooked ravioli. Pepper to taste and reheat.

- Sprinkle the ravioli with parmesan and serve with Grilled Vegetables (pg 72).

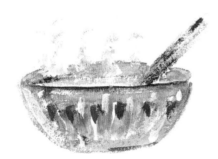

VARIATION

- Use linguine and add canned clams and pepper flakes for *á la Vongole* version of this dish.

Tortellini with Ratatouille Sauce

Pasta is the harassed cook's best friend as it blends with many flavors.

1 pkg	(454 g)	frozen cheese tortellini
500 ml	(2 cups)	ratatouille (commercial or see pg 67)
15 ml	(1 Tbsp)	oil
		salt and pepper
		grated parmesan

In a large saucepan of salted boiling water, cook the tortellini until al dente. Drain and return to the saucepan.

Add the ratatouille and oil and mix well. Salt and pepper to taste and reheat.

Sprinkle with parmesan and serve immediately.

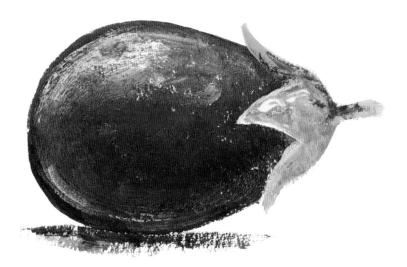

TIP
- While draining the pasta, save 250 to 500 ml (1-2 cups) of cooking water, which is rich in starch. When the pasta is cooked, mix with the sauce and add cooking water to adjust the consistency if needed.

VARIATION
- Garnish with sliced black olives.

Clam Linguine

Spaghettini, vermicelli, capelli d'angelo...any long pasta may be used in this recipe.

Preparation: 5 min Cooking time: 10 min Servings: 7

1 pkg	(500 g)	linguine
30 ml	(2 Tbsp)	oil
3		garlic cloves, slivered
2 cans	(284 ml/ 10 oz ea.)	small clams, with juice
125 ml	(1/2 cup)	white wine or water
		pepper
50 ml	(1/4 cup)	bread crumbs
45 ml	(3 Tbsp)	fresh parsley, finely chopped

In a large pot of salted boiling water, cook the pasta until al dente. Drain and keep warm.

Meanwhile, in a large non-stick skillet, heat 15 ml (1 Tbsp) oil on medium. Cook the garlic for 1-2 minutes (don't brown). Add the clams and their juice and the wine. Let simmer 2 minutes. Pepper to taste. Remove from heat.

In a small pan, heat the remaining oil on medium. Add the bread crumbs and sauté 2-3 minutes until golden. Stir in the parsley.

Combine the cooked pasta and clam sauce. Stir over heat until well heated. Add the seasonings. Divide the pasta on dinner plates and garnish with the bread crumbs. Serve immediately.

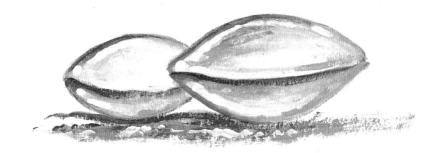

VARIATIONS

- Replace the clams with shrimp, and add approximately 125 ml (1/2 cup) of the pasta cooking water as a substitute for the clam juice.

- For a "shrimp and clam" version, replace one of the cans of clams with 225 g (1/2 lb) cooked Nordic shrimp.

- For a special occasion, add some fresh clams in the shell.

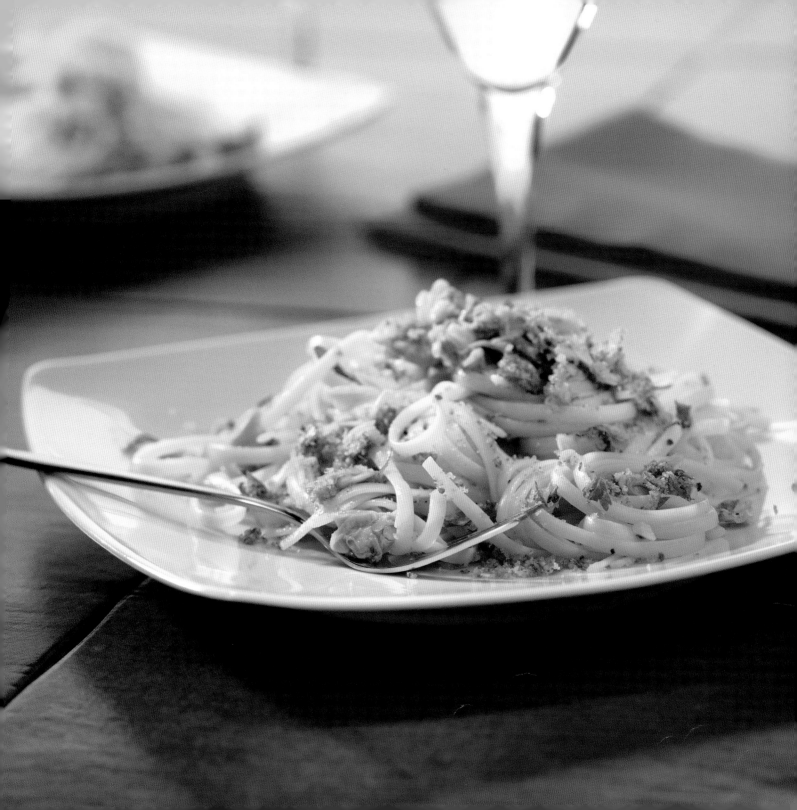

Vegetarian

Crispy Tofu

Daily consumption of soy products can lower blood cholesterol and fight osteoporosis in menopausal women.

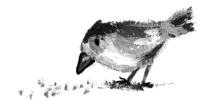

Preparation: 10 min Cooking time: 15 min Servings: 4 — **Vegetarian**

125 ml	(1/2 cup)	sesame seeds
5 ml	(1 tsp)	ground ginger
5 ml	(1 tsp)	chili powder
5 ml	(1 tsp)	ground coriander
5 ml	(1 tsp)	cumin
2 ml	(1/2 tsp)	salt
1 pkg	(454 g/16 oz)	extra firm tofu
15 ml	(1 Tbsp)	oil
45 ml	(3 Tbsp)	mirin or sweand wine
45 ml	(3 Tbsp)	water

- In a small bowl, mix the sesame seeds, ginger, chili powder, coriander, cumin and salt. Transfer to a shallow dish.

- Drain and wipe the tofu. Cut lengthwise into 6 slices of approximately 1 cm (1/2") thick. Coat each side of the tofu slices with the sesame and spice mixture. Reserve remaining spice mixture.

- In a non-stick skillet, heat oil on medium high. Fry the tofu slices 5 minutes or until they are golden and crisp. Turn and cook 5 more minutes.

- Mix the mirin and water. Pour into the skillet and stir to coat the tofu slices. The liquid will boil and evaporate quickly.

- Serve immediately with Chinese rice noodles or steamed rice and Tomato and Cucumber Salad (pg 68) and garnish with the sesame and spice mixture, if desired.

MY CHILD CAN...

- Prepare the spice mixture.
- Coat the tofu slices in the spice mixture.

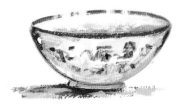

TIP

- Firm or extra firm tofu is ideal for this recipe. It is sold vacuum packed surrounded by water which you must wipe off in order to help the tofu absorb other flavors well. To do this, cut the tofu as indicated in the recipe, place it on two sheets of paper towels and cover with two more paper towels. To extract liquid, create pressure by placing unopened cans on the paper toweling for approximately 20 minutes.

Mozzarella *Carrozza*

A literal translation of this dish is "mozzarella in the car." It's a grilled mozzarella sandwich.

250 ml	(1 cup)	grated mozzarella
30 ml	(2 Tbsp)	mayonnaise
15 ml	(1 Tbsp)	Dijon mustard
15 ml	(1 Tbsp)	drained capers
		pepper
8		slices whole wheat bread
3		eggs
200 ml	(3/4 cup)	milk
75 ml	(1/3 cup)	flour
1 pinch		cayenne
10 ml	(2 tsp)	oil

Preheat the broiler.

In a bowl, mix the mozzarella, mayonnaise, Dijon mustard and capers. Pepper to taste. Spread 4 slices of bread with this mixture and top with the remaining 4 slices.

In a small bowl, mix the eggs and milk. In another bowl, mix the flour and cayenne. Dip each side of the sandwich in the egg mixture and land excess drip into the bowl. Coat each side in the flour mixture and dip once again in the egg mixture.

In a large ovenproof pan, preferably cast iron, heat 5 ml (1 tsp) oil on medium. Cook 2 sandwiches at once, without turning, for 2 minutes, or until the bottom is golden.

Place the pan under the broiler until they puff and are golden. Repeat with the other 2 sandwiches.

Serve with a crispy green salad.

MY CHILD CAN...

- Grate the cheese.
- Prepare the flour mixture.
- Dip the sandwiches in the egg mix and cot them with flour.

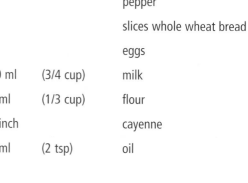

VARIATION

- Stir a little grated zucchini into the mozzarella mixture. To absorb any excess liquid from the zucchini, pat gently in a tea towel.

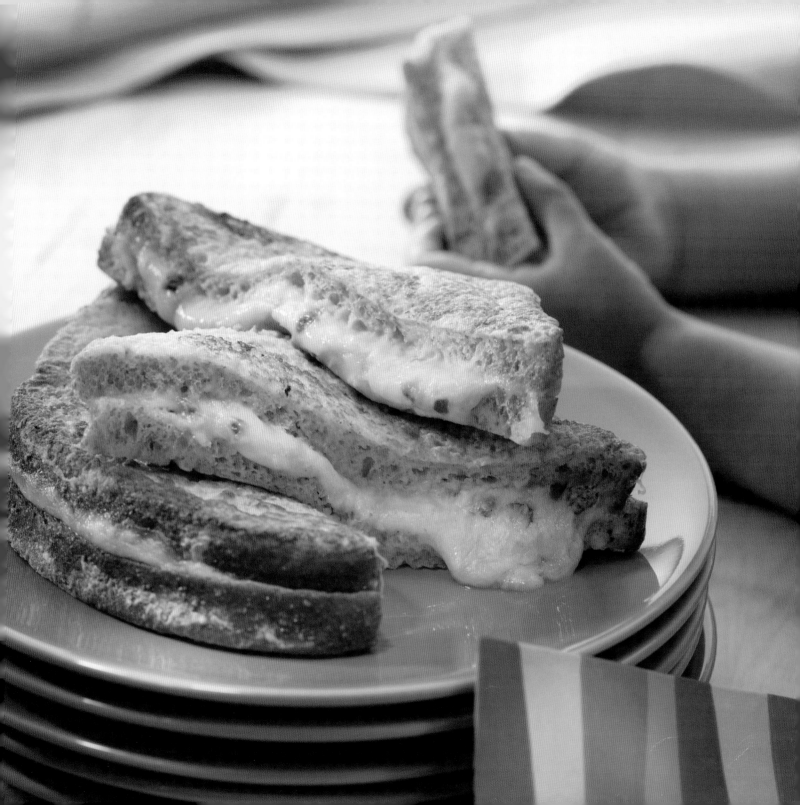

East Indian Chick Peas

Today's cuisine is exciting as we travel the world from home!
This recipe lands us taste the typical flavors and aromas of India.

Preparation: 10 min Cooking time: 25 min Servings: 5

**Vegetarian
Can be frozen**

3		cloves garlic
1 piece		fresh ginger, peeled (4 cm/1 1/2 in long)
1		large onion, quartered
15 ml	(1 Tbsp)	oil
15 ml	(1 Tbsp)	curry
15 ml	(1 Tbsp)	cumin
2		potatoes, peeled and diced (preferably Yukon Gold)
375 ml	(1 1/2 cup)	water
50 ml	(1/4 cup)	currants
		salt
1 boîte	(540 ml/19 oz)	chick peas, rinsed and drained
200 ml	(3/4 cup)	frozen green peas
		whole wheat pitas

Using a food processor or a hand-held blender, purée the ginger and garlic. Add the onion and pulse the processor to rough-chop the onion.

In a large skillet, heat the oil on medium and sauté the onion mixture, while stirring, 10 minutes or until lightly golden. Stir in the spices.

Add the potatoes, water and currants. Salt to taste and simmer 10 minutes or until the potatoes are cooked.

Stir in the chick peas and green peas. Cover and continue cooking 5 minutes or until the green peas are cooked.

Serve with heated pitas and garnish with Garlic and Mint Yogurt Sauce (pg 69).

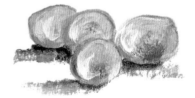

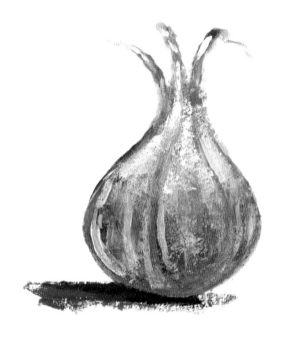

- Peel the ginger and/or the potatoes.
- Rinse the chick peas.

TIPS

- If you don't have currants, use chopped Sultana raisins.
- To avoid potatoes becoming green and bitter, store them away from light. Storing potatoes in too warm a temperature will cause germination, while storing them in too cold a temperature will cause them to develop a sweet taste which will cause them to darken when cooked. Only new potatoes should be stored in the refrigerator.

VARIATION

- Serve the chick pea mixture on a bed of basmati rice.

Mushroom, Spinach and Feta Barley

Barley can easily replace rice in any recipe, even risottos, as this version will demonstrate.

Preparation: 10 min Cooking time: 40 min Servings: 5

**Vegetarian
Can be frozen**

10 ml	(2 tsp)	oil
1		chopped onion
500 ml	(2 cups)	sliced mushrooms
125 ml	(1/2 cup)	frozen spinach (8 nuggands)
2		garlic cloves chopped
250 ml	(1 cup)	pearl barley
500 ml	(2 cups)	chicken or vegetable stock
125 ml	(1/2 cup)	crumbled feta
30 ml	(2 Tbsp)	lemon juice
		salt and pepper

- In a large saucepan, heat 5 ml (1 tsp) oil on medium and sauté the onions, mushrooms, spinach and garlic for 8 minutes or until the onion is soft and the spinach defrosted. Set aside.

- In the same saucepan, heat the remaining oil and sauté the barley until it is coated with oil.

- Add the stock and bring to the boil. Reduce the heat, cover and let simmer 10-30 minutes until the barley is cooked.

- Stir in the cooked vegetables, feta and lemon juice. Salt and pepper to taste. Let rest a few minutes before serving.

MY CHILD CAN...

- Crumble the feta.
- Juice the lemon.

TIP

- To shorten preparation time, buy pre-sliced mushrooms.

VARIATIONS

- Add some cooked bacon bits.
- Add some cooked, cleaned shrimp.
- Add cooked merguez or chorizo in bite size pieces.

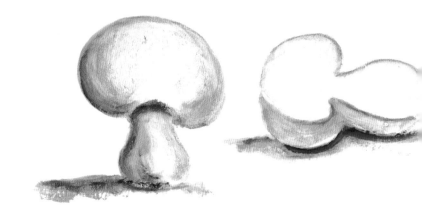

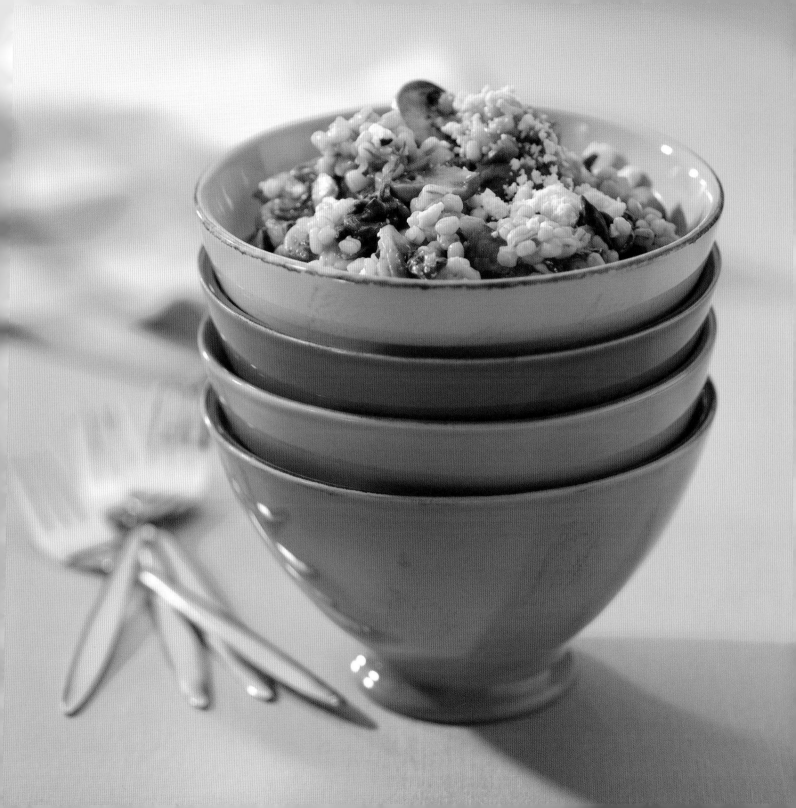

Eggs

Broccoli Frittata

For a light supper, serve this frittata with a green salad or the Tomato and Cucumber Salad (pg 68). The frittata can also be cut in wedges and served as an hors d'oeuvre.

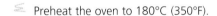

Preparation: 15 min Baking time: 30 min Servings: 6

10 ml	(2 tsp)	oil
30 ml	(2 Tbsp)	bread crumbs
125 ml	(1/2 cup)	grated old cheddar
4		eggs
250 ml	(1 cup)	milk
10 ml	(2 tsp)	Dijon mustard
1 ml	(1/4 tsp)	salt
750 ml	(3 cups)	broccoli florets
90 g	(3 oz)	sliced back bacon cubed

Preheat the oven to 180°C (350°F).

Lightly oil the bottom and sides of a 23 cm (9") diameter pie plate. Coat the bottom and sides of the pie plate with the bread crumbs. Place the cheese in the bottom of the pie plate. Set aside.

In a large bowl, mix the eggs, milk, mustard and salt. Set aside.

Cook the broccoli until tender. Cool in cold water, drain and chop coarsely. Set aside.

In a skillet, fry the bacon until crisp. Stir the broccoli and bacon bits into the egg mixture. Pour into the prepared pie plate.

Bake 30 minutes or until the top of the frittata is browned.

Let cool slightly and serve.

MY CHILD CAN...

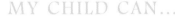

- Prepare the pie plate.
- Mix the eggs, milk, mustard and salt.

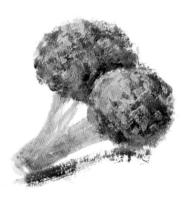

TIP
- Store eggs in their original container, since the shell is porous and absorbs odors. Also, don't store them in the door shelf since the temperature fluctuates here.

VARIATION
- Replace the back bacon with diced smoked bacon.

Eggs à La Carte

Low on inspiration and time? Here is a meal to please everyone.
And they get to choose their own toppings. A perfect meal for Sunday brunch!

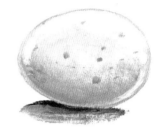

Preparation: 15 min Baking time: 10 min Servings: 6

6		slices of bread 2 cm (3/4 in) thick
15 ml	(1 Tbsp)	butter
6		eggs
		pepper

- Preheat the oven to 200°C (400°F).
- Butter one side of each slice of bread. Place them, buttered side down, on a parchment-lined baking sheet.
- With your fingers, make a dent in the center of each slice by crushing the bread down.
- Break an egg into each center without breaking the yolk. Add one of the suggested toppings. Pepper to taste.
- Cook 10 minutes or until the cheese melts and the egg is almost cooked.
- Serve with a mesclun salad.

TOPPING IDEAS
(for one serving)

- **Ham and Cheese**
  A slice of ham and about 30 ml (2 Tbsp) grated gruyère cheese.
- **Asparagus - Old Cheddar**
  Two cooked asparagus spears cut in chunks, and approximately 30 ml (2 Tbsp) grated old cheddar.
- **Tomato - Parmesan**
  One sliced plum tomato and approximately 30 ml (2 Tbsp) grated parmesan.
- **Bacon - Blue Cheese**
  One or two slices of cooked back bacon, diced and approximately 30 ml (2 Tbsp) crumbled blue cheese.
- **Mushroom - Emmenthal**
  Two finely sliced mushrooms and approximately 30 ml (2 Tbsp) grated emmenthal.

MY CHILD CAN...

- Butter the slices of bread.
- Crush the centre of each slice of bread.
- Choose and prepare his own topping.

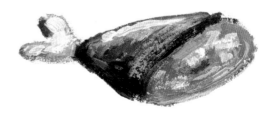

TIP

- To confirm the doneness of the egg, gently shake the baking sheet. The eggs should jiggle. The eggs will continue to cook when removed from the oven.

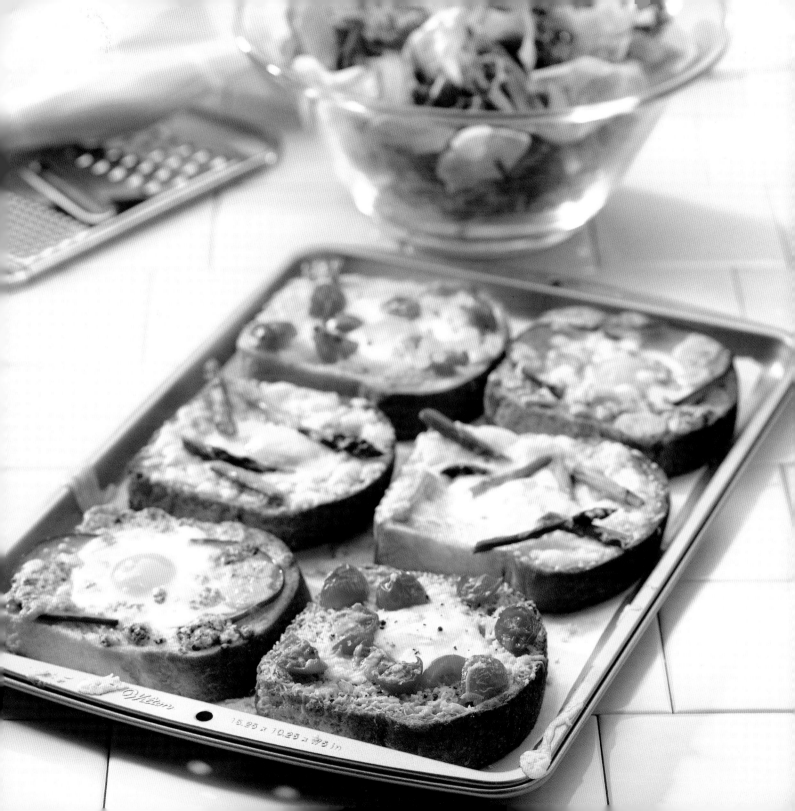

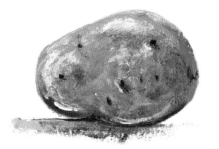

Potato **Frittata**

You can very successfully prepare frittata in advance. It can be a main meal or an hors d'oeuvre either at room temperature or slightly heated.

Preparation: 15 min Cooking time: 25 min Servings: 5   **Vegetarian**

15 ml	(3 tsp)	oil
2		medium potatoes, halved, thinly sliced
2		large onions, halved, thinly sliced
30 ml	(2 Tbsp)	fresh chopped chives or 10 ml (2 tsp) dried chives
5 ml	(1 tsp)	salt
		pepper
6		eggs
45 ml	(3 Tbsp)	fresh chopepd parsley

In a large non-stick ovenproof skillet heat 10 ml (2 tsp) oil on medium, and sauté the potatoes, onions and chives. Shake on 2 ml (1/2 tsp) salt.

Cook, stirring occasionally, for 5 minutes or until the vegetables are soft and browned. Transfer to a large bowl, pepper to taste and leave to cool slightly.

In another bowl, beat the eggs with the parsley. Stir in the remaining salt. Pour over the lukewarm vegetables and mix well.

In the same skillet, heat the remaining 5 ml (1 tsp) oil on medium high. Pour the mixture of egg and vegetables into the bottom of the pan. Cook 5 minutes or until the potatoes are golden.

Place the oven rack approximately 15 cm (6") away from the preheated broiler.

Cover the skillet handle with a double layer of aluminum foil to prevent it burning under the broiler.

Place the skillet under the broiler for 2 minutes or until the frittata is cooked to the center.

Slip the frittata on a platter and let it rest a few minutes. Cut and serve with a spinach salad.

MY CHILD CAN...

- Crack open the eggs.

- Cut the potatoes and onions under the supervision of an adult.

VARIATION

- Use approximately 500 ml (2 cups) of previously prepared and frozen Mexican Roast Vegetables (pg 121), stir in the egg mixture and cook in the same fashion.

Greek Quiche

Prepare two quiche at the same time. Once they are cooked, you may freeze one of them.

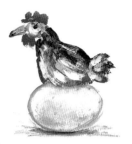

Preparation: 15 min Baking time: 30 min Servings: 5

**Vegetarian
Can be frozen**

5 ml	(1 tsp)	oil
1		small chopped onion
1		pie shell 23 cm (9 in) diameter, uncooked
1 can	(398 ml/14 oz)	artichokes, drained, quartered and patted dry
50 ml	(1/4 cup)	frozen chopped spinach, defrosted, well drained (or 5 muggets)
90 g	(3 oz)	crumbled feta
4		eggs
125 ml	(1/2 cup)	milk
1 ml	(1/4 tsp)	fennel seeds
		pepper
50 ml	(1/4 cup)	sliced black olives

- Preheat the oven to 190°C (375°F).

- In a small pan, heat oil and sauté the onion 5 minutes or until they are tender. Set aside.

- Arrange the artichoke quarters on the bottom of the pie crust.

- Mix the cooked onion, spinach, feta, eggs, milk and fennel seeds. Pepper to taste.

- Pour the egg mixture over the contents in the pie crust. Garnish with the sliced black olives.

- Place the quiche on a baking sheet and bake 30 minutes or until the top is golden.

- Serve with fresh tomato quarters.

MY CHILD CAN...

- Crack open the eggs.
- Quarter the artichokes.
- Drain the spinach and crumble the feta.

TIP

- For a drier and flakier pie crust, place the pie, pastry or quiche on a baking sheet, especially if it is an aluminum pie plate, and place in the oven.

VARIATIONS

- Omit the pastry crust and proceed, following the instruction for Broccoli Frittata (pg 161).
- For a more sophisticated version, replace the pie pastry with rolled puff pastry or fillo pastry.

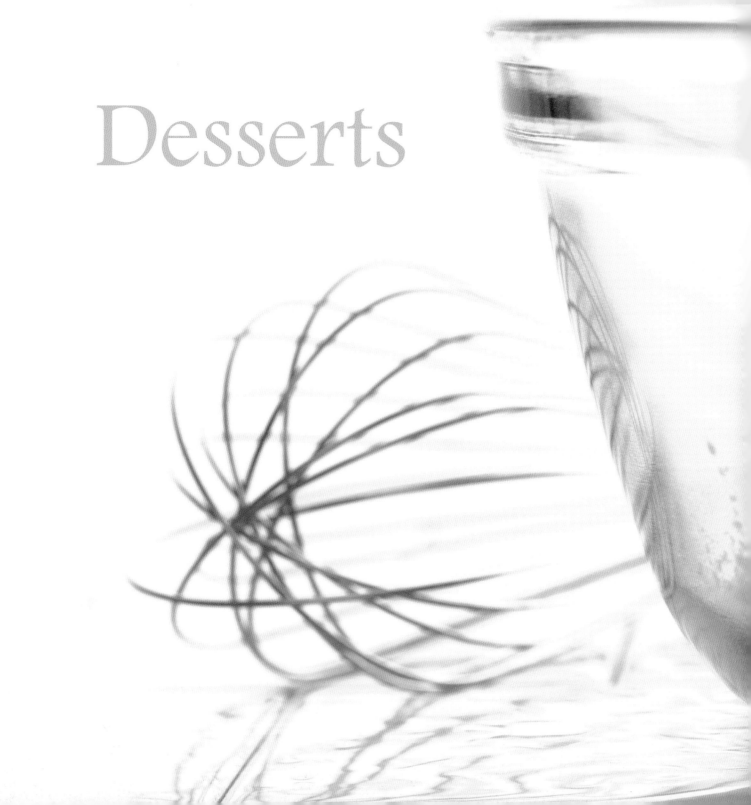

Desserts

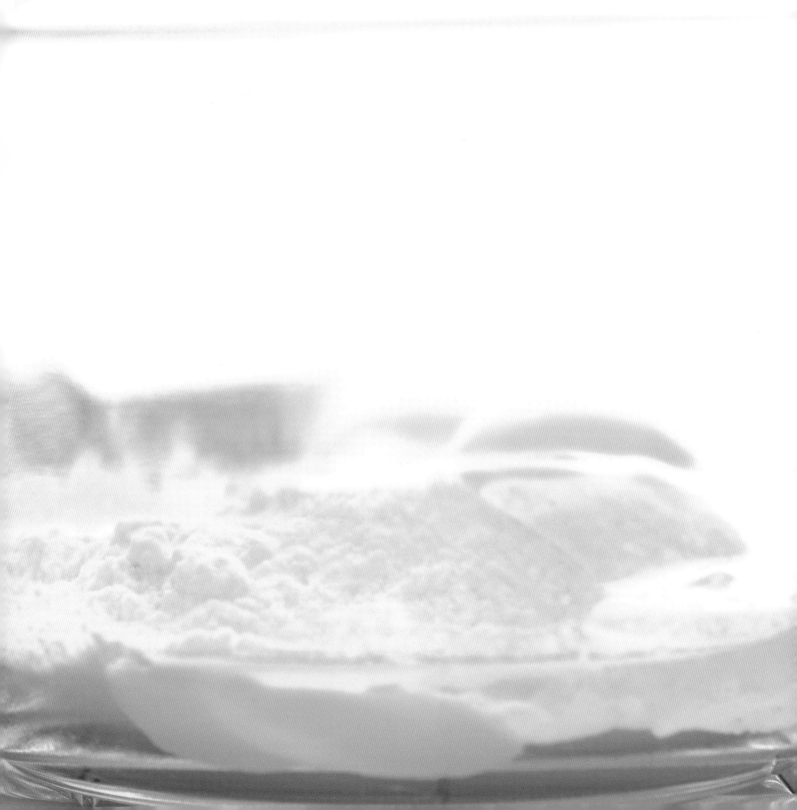

Fresh Cheese **Crêpes**

Mouth-watering crêpes filled with a creamy smooth filling. How could you resist?

Preparation: 20 min Baking time: 10 min Servings: 4

Can be frozen
(without filling)

CRÊPES

200 ml	(3/4 cup)	flour
250 ml	(1 cup)	milk
2		eggs
15 ml	(1 Tbsp)	sugar
5 ml	(1 tsp)	vanilla
1 ml	(1/4 tsp)	salt

FILLING

3 mini containers 60 g (each)		fresh cheese (i.e. Danone)
		apple sauce or some peaches

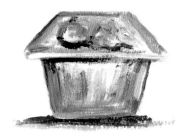

In the bowl of the food processor, mix all crêpe ingredients until thoroughly mixed. Transfer to a bowl.

Lightly oil the bottom of a non-stick 15 cm (6") pan and heat on medium. Pour approximately 60 ml (4 Tbsp) of crêpe batter into pan, turning to evenly cover the bottom.

Cook approximately 30 seconds or until the bottom of the crêpe is golden. Without flipping the crêpe to cook the top, place on a plate. Repeat the procedure with the remaining batter and stack the cooked crêpes. Makes 12 crêpes.

Preheat the oven to 190°C (375°F).

Lightly oil a 23 x 33 cm (19" x 13") baking dish.

Place a 15 ml (1 Tbsp) dollop of fresh cheese in the center of each crêpe. Fold the top and the bottom to the center and then fold in the sides.

Arrange the crêpes, folded side down, in the prepared dish. (You could prepare crêpes to this point, cover them, and refrigerate until the next day.)

Cook 10 minutes or until a knife inserted into the center of the crêpe comes out hot. Serve with apple sauce or peaches.

MY CHILD CAN...
* Fill and fold the crêpes.

VARIATION
* Eat the crêpes hot with cold fresh cheese for a contrast in temperature.

The Smoothy

For breakfast, or to satisfy an afternoon craving, there is nothing like this nutritious drink. Discovers the wonders of probiotic yogurts. Probiotics, especially those with a lactobacillus base, contribute to the healthy functioning of the digestive system (see pg 47). Enjoy it every day.

Preparation: 5 min Servings: 2

250 ml	(1 cup)	milk
125 ml	(1/2 cup)	orange juice
125 ml	(1/2 cup)	vanilla probiotic yogurt (i.e. Activia)
30 ml	(2 Tbsp)	powdered milk
15 ml	(1 Tbsp)	chocolate milk powder

In the blender or with a hand-held mixer, blend the ingredients to a smooth purée. Enjoy.

MY CHILD CAN...

- Prepare her own Smoothy, under adult supervision (make sure that the blender lid is closed).

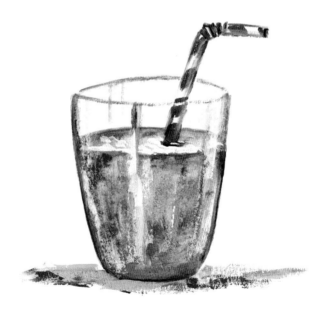

VARIATIONS

- For extra fiber, add 15 ml (1 Tbsp) oat bran per 250 ml (1 cup) serving.
- For extra omega 3, add 5 ml (1 tsp) flax seed oil per 250 ml (1 cup) serving.

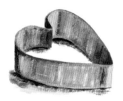

Decorator **Cake** Delight

What can be more fun than everyone decorating their own piece of cake...with candy!

Preparation: 15 min Baking time: 30 min Servings: 10   **Can be Frozen**

125 ml	(1/2 cup)	flour
125 ml	(1/2 cup)	whole wheat flour
125 ml	(1/2 cup)	cocoa powder
2 ml	(1/2 tsp)	salt
75 ml	(1/3 cup)	chocolate chips
300 ml	(1 1/4 cup)	light brown sugar, packed
50 ml	(1/4 cup)	canola oil
50 ml	(1/4 cup)	plain yogurt or buttermilk
2		eggs
10 ml	(2 tsp)	vanilla
10 containers 60 g		fresh cheese (i.e. Danone)
		a variety of candy

Preheat oven to 180°C (350°F).

Lightly oil a square 23 cm (9") dish and powder with flour. Set aside.

In a small bowl, beat the brown sugar, oil, yogurt, eggs and vanilla until the mixture is well combined. Mix in the dry ingredients and the chocolate chips, stirring just until the dry ingredients are moistened.

Pour into the prepared cake pan. Bake 30 minutes or until a toothpick inserted in the center of the cake comes out clean.

Let cool and cut into varied sized servings.

Serve with a mini container of fresh cheese and offer various candies for each guest to decorate their own individualized creation!

MY CHILD CAN...

- Test the freshness of the chocolate chips during the preparation of the cake...

- Decorate his cake however he wants.

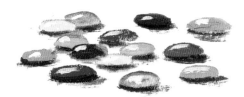

VARIATIONS

- For a "chicken feed" look, use white chocolate chips.
- For a refreshing cool dessert, freeze the 60 g fresh cheese containers and serve them frozen.
- For an amusing version, use many different shapes: circles, diamonds, hearts...

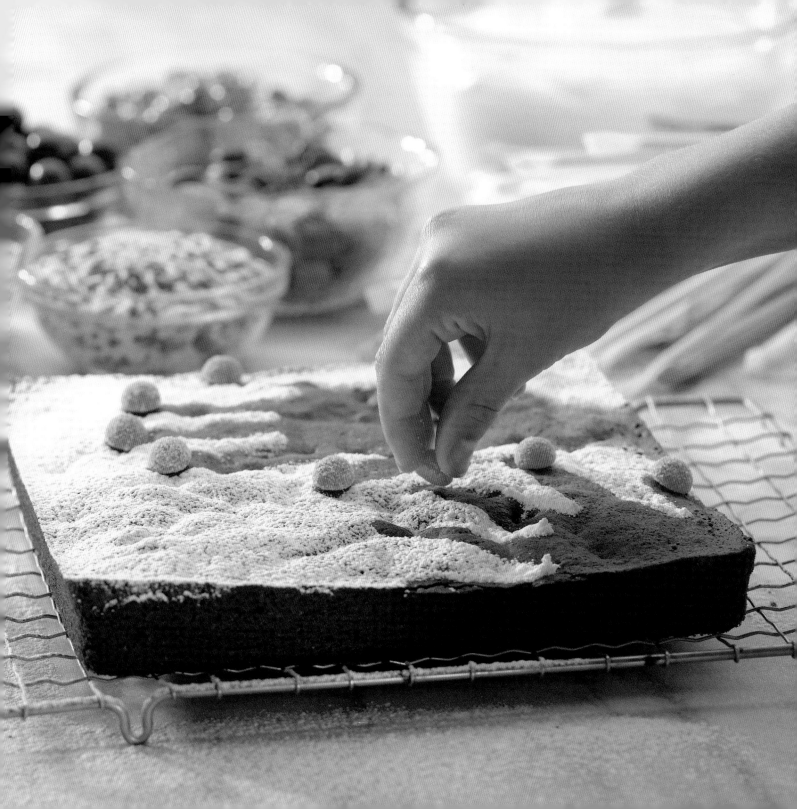

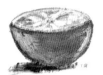

Date and Orange Squares

These are favorites as a snack or a dessert; they are even better warmed and are guaranteed to contain no trans fats.

Preparation: 20 min Baking time: 30 min Servings: 16   **Can be frozen**

500 g	(1 lb)	pitted dried dates
1		large orange, peeled, cut into small pieces
125 ml	(1/2 cup)	orange juice
375 ml	(1 1/2 cup)	old fashioned rolled oats
375 ml	(1 1/2 cup)	flour
250 ml	(1 cup)	light brown sugar, lightly packed
2 ml	(1/2 tsp)	salt
125 ml	(1/2 cup)	canola oil
50 ml	(1/4 cup)	melted butter

Preheat the oven to 180°C (350°F).

Mix the dates, orange pieces and juice in a small saucepan. Cover and cook 10 minutes on medium or until the dates are soft. Crush them with the back of a spoon, breaking them into pieces. Set aside.

In a bowl, mix the rolled oats, flour, brown sugar and salt. Beat in the butter and oil.

Press half of this oat mixture on the bottom of a 23 cm (9") square baking dish. Spread the date mixture over this. Sprinkle the remaining oat mixture on top of dates.

Bake 30 minutes or until the top is golden.

Cool and cut into 16 squares.

DID YOU KNOW...

- Rolled oats retain a good part of the germ and bran (outer cover) of the grain during processing, making this a nutritious ceral rich in fibre. it doesn't matter which rolled oats you buy, they are all made from the entire grain.

MY CHILD CAN...

- Measure the dry ingredients.
- Prepare the oat mixture.
- Cut the orange with an appropriate knife under adult supervision.

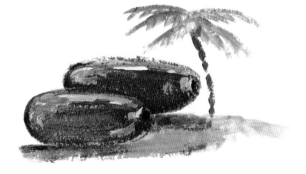

Raspberry Cream

Filled with good soy phytoestrogens, this devilishly easy-to-prepare dessert is divinely delicious.

Preparation: 10 min (Waiting Time 30 min) Servings: 6

1 pkg	(340 g/12 oz)	silken tofu
30 ml	(2 Tbsp)	maple syrup
250 ml	(1 cup)	raspberries, fresh or frozen
5 ml	(1 tsp)	vanilla
		fresh mint leaves (optional)
		fresh raspberries (optional)

In the jar of a blender or with a hand-held mixer, blend all ingredients to a smooth purée.

Pour into individual serving dishes. Refrigerate at least 30 minutes before serving.

Garnish with mint leaves and a few fresh raspberries, if desired.

DID YOU KNOW...

- Commercial jelled food sets much faster than homemade jelled food. It therefore keeps in more flavour, texture and nutritive value.

MY CHILD CAN...

- Prepare the cream under adult supervision and pour it into dessert dishes.

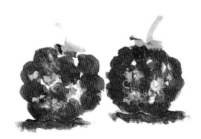

VARIATION

- Replace the raspberries with fresh or frozen strawberries or canned pears.

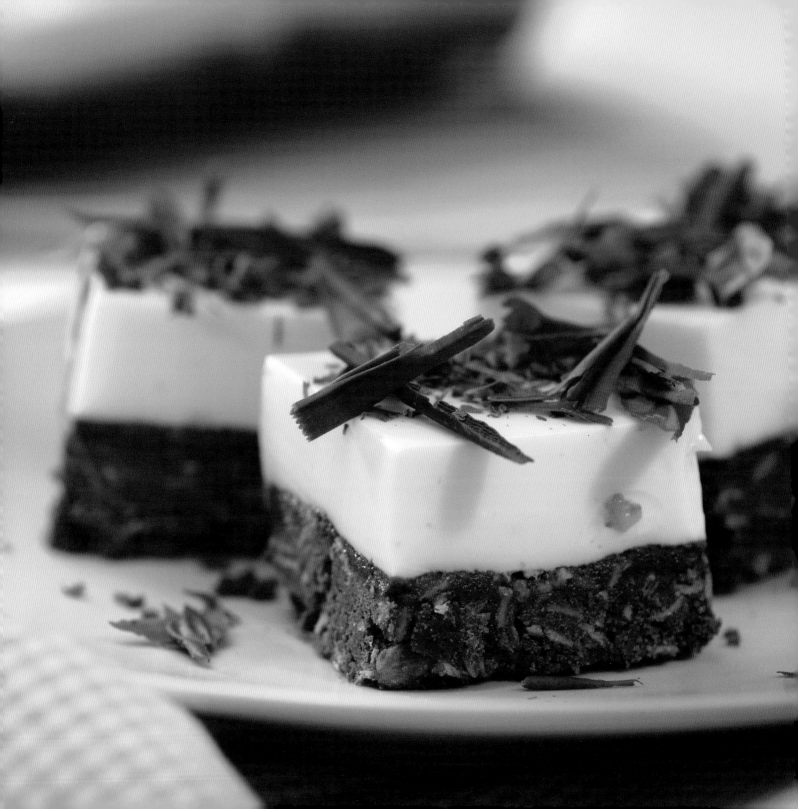

Pear Yogurt Squares

Elegant enough to serve to guests but simple enough to serve on a week day.

Preparation: 15 min Baking time: 10 min Servings: 12
(SETTING TIME: 1 H 30)

CRUST

375 ml	(1 1/2 cup)	flour
250 ml	(1 cup)	rolled oats
250 ml	(1 cup)	brown sugar
45 ml	(3 Tbsp)	cocoa powder
5 ml	(1 tsp)	ground cinnamon
2 ml	(1/2 tsp)	salt
125 ml	(1/2 cup)	canola oil
3 squares	(100 g/3 oz)	bitter-sweet chocolate, melted

GARNISH

1 1/2 enveloppe		plain gelatin
1 pot	(650 g)	probiotic pear yogurt (i.e. Activia)

Preheat oven to 180°C (350°F).

In a bowl, mix the flour, rolled oats, brown sugar, cocoa, cinnamon and salt. Add the oil and the chocolate and mix well. Press this mixture with your fingers into the bottom of a 30 x 20 cm (12" x 8") baking dish. Bake 10 minutes. Let cool.

In a small bowl, dissolve the gelatin in 125 ml (1/2 cup) cold water for a few minutes.

In a thick bottomed saucepan or in the microwave, melt the gelatin completely to obtain a liquid gelatin, but don't overheat. Stir in the yogurt.

Pour the yogurt preparation on the cooled crust. Refrigerate at least one hour before serving.

Cut into 12 squares and accompany with pear slices, chocolate sauce or simply garnish with chocolate curls.

This will keep refrigerated for 5 days.

MY CHILD CAN...

- Finger press the oat mixture into the bottom of the baking dish.

VARIATION

- Replace the pear yogurt with any other flavor of probiotic yogurt that you like.

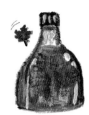

Maple Pudding

More nourishing and tasty than those little containers of commercial pudding!

Preparation: 5 min Cooking time: 10 min Servings: 6
(SETTING TIME 30 MIN)

2		eggs
60 ml	(4 Tbsp)	corn starch
125 ml	(1/2 cup)	maple syrup
500 ml	(2 cups)	milk
		maple syrup (optional)

In a thick bottomed saucepan, mix the eggs, corn starch and maple syrup until smooth and the corn starch is completely dissolved. Add the milk while beating with a whisk. Cook on medium stirring constantly until thick.

Pour into individual dessert dishes. Refrigerate at least 30 minutes. At the moment of serving, top with maple syrup, if desired.

MY CHILD CAN...

- Cook the pudding under adult supervision and pour into the dessert bowls.

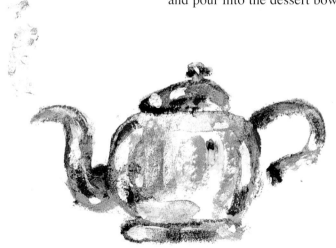

TIP
- Use this pudding to fill a Boston cream pie. You could use the pudding as the center filling of a vanilla cake and top it with softened chocolate ice cream.

Fruit Variations

So many simple ways to eat fruit!

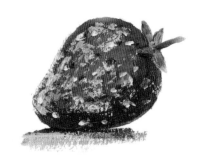

TROPICAL FRUIT

Preparation: 5 min

Serve pineapple, mango and/or papaya slices with vanilla probiotic yogurt and sprinkle with toasted coconut.

ICED LITCHIS

Preparation: 5 min (Setting time 2 h)

For an original frozen treat, drain canned litchi fruit, freeze on a baking sheet for at least 2 hours, then serve in a champagne flute.

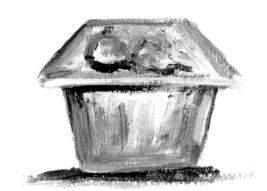

VANILLA APPLES

Preparation: 10 min Cooking time: 5 min Servings: 4

In a large skillet, heat 250 ml (1 cup) of water with 75 ml (1/3 cup) brown sugar and 5 ml (1 tsp) vanilla until the sugar is dissolved. Meanwhile, peel (or not) 2 apples and slice them into wedges. Place the apple slices in the syrup and simmer 5 minutes or until they are tender. Serve with a bit of the syrup and also apple muesli probiotic yogurt (i.e. Activia).

HOMEMADE JELL~O

Preparation: 10 min (Setting time 1 h) Servings: 5

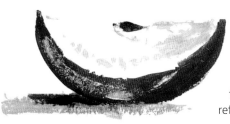

In a large bowl, sprinkle an envelope of unflavored gelatin on 50 ml (1/2 cup) cold water and let dissolve 1 minute. Mix 15 ml (1 Tbsp) sugar with 125 ml (1/2 cup) boiling white grape juice and then pour into the gelatin mixture to dissolve it. Add 250 ml (1 cup) cold grape juice. Divide 250 ml (1 cup) small chunks of fresh fruit or frozen fruit into 125 ml (1/2 cup) glass ramekins. Pour the fruit juice mixture over the fruit, refrigerate, and let set for at least 1 hour.

Fruit Variations

VANILLA APPLE SAUCE

Preparation: 10 min Cooking time: 10 min Servings: 3

Peel and slice 6 apples. Place the slices in a large microwave proof glass bowl. Stir in 50 ml (1/4 cup) water or apple juice, 50 ml (1/4 cup) brown sugar and 10 ml (2 tsp) vanilla. Cover and cook on high for 4 minutes. Stir and cook 3 minutes longer or until the apples are soft. Serve as is, warm or cold, or mash with a potato masher.

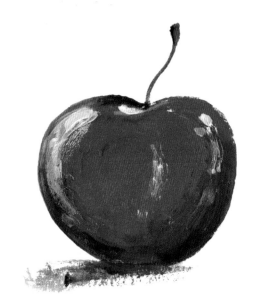

GRILLED FRUIT

Preparation: 5 min Baking Time: 15 min Servings: 6

Preheat oven to 220°C (425°F). Halve 2 apples, 2 pears and 2 plums, pit and core them and arrange the fruit, cut side up, in a shallow baking dish. Sprinkle the fruit with 30 ml (2 Tbsp) sugar and cardamom, cinnamon and ground nutmeg, to taste. Bake 15 minutes or just until the sugar begins to caramelize. Serve with frozen vanilla yogurt or vanilla probiotic yogurt. (i.e. Activia)

TROPICAL SHERBERT

Preparation: 5 min (Setting time 30 min) Servings: 8

In a blender or food processor, combine 750 ml (3 cups) frozen tropical fruit and 75 ml (1/3 cup) sugar and pulse to coarse chop. While the processor is running, add 200 ml (3/4 cup) natural probiotic yogurt, and 15 ml (1 Tbsp) orange juice. Spoon into fruit bowls. Put in the freezer for 15-30 minutes and serve. (If the sherbert is frozen more than 2 hours, it will be very hard and you will need to purée it in a food processor to give it a smooth texture.) Garnish with mint leaves.

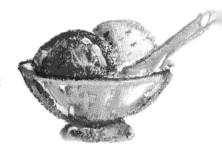

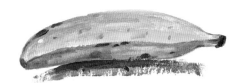

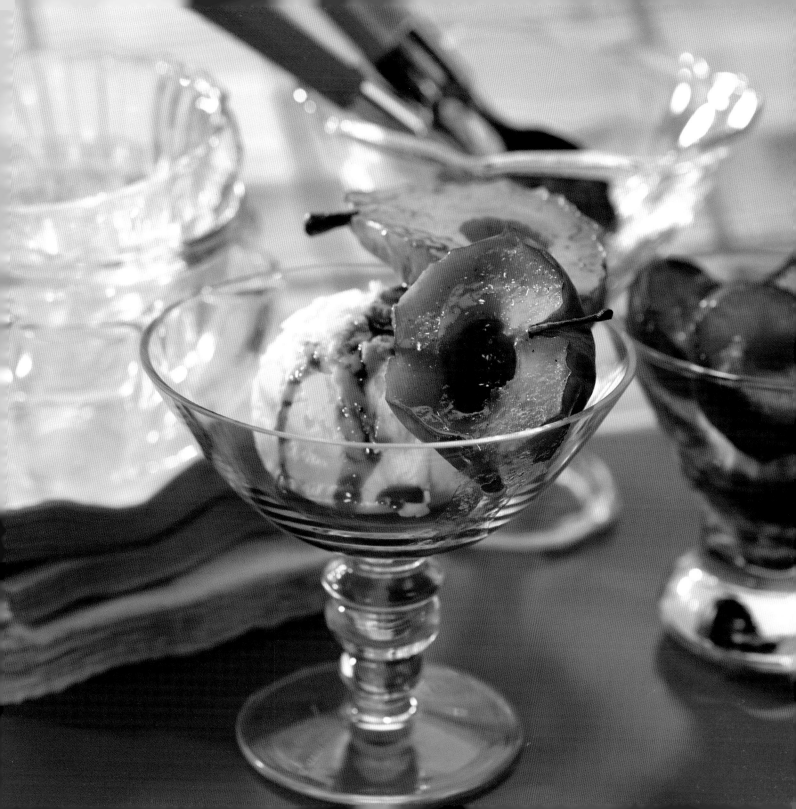

Nutritional Values

Each recipe has been analyzed to provide nutritional values per serving, whether in calories, protein, sugars, fiber, fat or sodium content. When a recipe lists its ingredients, it is the first ingredient which is selected and analyzed for its nutritional value. The following, unless otherwise indicated, are various ingredients we used in the recipes and upon which we based our nutritional analysis.

180

Milk and yogurt:	1% milk, 1% yogurt
Evaporated milk:	partly skimmed evaporated milk
Mozzarella:	partly skimmed mozzarella
Parmesan:	fresh grated parmesan (for the taste)
Eggs:	large size
Oil:	olive oil
Flour:	All purpose
Ground beef:	lean ground beef
Soy sauce:	light soy sauce

Recipes	Per Serving	Calories	Protein (g)	Sugar (g)	Fiber (g)	Fat (g)	Sodium (mg)
Basic Recipes and Accompaniments							
Creamed Corn Soup	300 ml	148	8.7	25	1.2	2.4	290
Roasted Root Vegetables	1 serving	156	2.6	27	4.6	4.9	570
Ratatouille	200 ml	87	2.8	15	3	2.8	27
Tomato and Cucumber Salad	200 ml	80	0.8	4.4	1.2	7.1	7.1
Garlic and Mint Yogurt Sauce	300 ml	21	1.7	2.5	0	0.5	134
Tomato Sauce	200 ml	84	4.6	14	4.9	3.5	836
White Sauce	125 ml	90	5.3	14	0.3	1.5	239

Recipes	Per Serving	Calories	Protein (g)	Sugar (g)	Fiber (g)	Fat (g)	Sodium (mg)
Vegetable Variations							181
Grilled Vegetables	1 serving	130	2.4	13	2.8	8.6	9.2
Fennel Salad	1 serving	77	1	11	1.1	3.7	26
Carrot Ribbons	1/2 carrot	30	0.5	4.8	1.1	1.2	15
Grilled Tomatoes	1 tomato	87	3	8.4	1.7	5.2	111
Soups – Main Courses							
Pasta and Chick Pea Soup	375 ml	298	16	47	7.4	7	963
Asian Tofu Soup	400 ml	316	21	40	2.8	9.2	992
Indian Lentil Soup	330 ml	232	17	36	6.9	3.1	408
Chicken Rice Soup	375 ml	181	18	21	0.8	2.4	721
Chicken and Bean Soup	300 ml	247	24	30	7.1	3.6	320
Italian Sausage Soup	330 ml	298	17	25	3.6	15	941
Beef							
Parmesan Meatballs	4 meatballs	220	19	2.9	0.3	14	159
Moroccan Style Pitas	1 pita	417	26	42	4.2	18	513
Sage Beef Stew	1 1/2 cups	243	27	10	2.7	9.3	196
Orange Beef Stir-Fry	1 serving	214	19	23	1.3	5.1	176
Grilled Beef Flank	100 g	205	25	1.9	0.2	10	45

Recipes	Per Serving	Calories	Protein (g)	Sugar (g)	Fiber (g)	Fat (g)	Sodium (mg)
Bolognaise Sauce	190 ml	296	25	11	1.9	14	97
Steak w/ Mushroom-Coffee Sauce	1 serving	206	27	6	0.9	8.3	179
Tex-Mex Tacos	1 taco	256	18	29	3.8	8.2	82

Veal

Rigatoni and Sausage Casserole	300 ml	452	24	56	5.3	15	744
Apple Veal Cutlets	1 cutlet	192	27	11	1.4	4.1	190
Hunter Veal Stew	250 ml	240	29	13	4.3	8.7	632
Veal Burgers and Mushrooms	1 burger	221	16	26	2.7	5	295

Pork

Pear and Ginger Pork Cutlets	100 g	215	24	13	1.1	7.1	250
Tomato Pesto Pork Cutlets	100 g	182	20	2	0.7	9.8	223
Maple Pork Tenderloin	100 g	221	30	14	0.2	3.9	356

Chicken

Chicken Enchiladas	1 enchilada	348	32	28	2.3	9.3	736
Chinese Chicken	1 serving	150	22	3.7	0.1	2.9	370
Chicken Cacciatore	1 chicken leg	293	30	12	3.5	14	305

Recipes	Per Serving	Calories	Protein (g)	Sugar (g)	Fiber (g)	Fat (g)	Sodium (mg)
Chicken Couscous	1 serving	260	24	25	5.3	7.7	309
Curry Chicken in Cream Sauce	1 serving	221	31	12	0.9	5	447
Chicken on Fennel	1 serving	236	25	15	2.4	8.6	396
Sesame Crusted Chicken Salad	1 serving	317	32	9.3	3.4	17	74
Four Step Chicken	1 serving	170	22	5.2	1.4	6.2	91
Mexican Roast Vegetables and Chicken	1 serving	347	27	37	5.2	11	272
Parmesan Chicken	1 serving	186	27	9.1	1.6	4.4	547

Turkey

Recipes	Per Serving	Calories	Protein (g)	Sugar (g)	Fiber (g)	Fat (g)	Sodium (mg)
Red Kidney Bean Chili	250 ml	300	23	23	5,3	11	84
Turkey Piccata	100 g	198	29	1.9	0.1	7.6	228
Mexican Macaroni	300 ml	249	15	37	5.1	5.4	379
Meat Loaf	1 slice	199	21	6	1.1	9.7	408
Asian Turkey Roll	1 roll	239	19	19	2.2	9.7	240

Fish

Recipes	Per Serving	Calories	Protein (g)	Sugar (g)	Fiber (g)	Fat (g)	Sodium (mg)
Tuna Croque-Monsieur	1 croque-m.	264	27	17	2.1	9.6	460
Asian Salmon Croquettes	1 croquette	127	17	6.8	0.7	3.7	170
Fish Fillets with Herb Sauce	125 g	225	28	0.6	0.2	11	151

Recipes	Per Serving	Calories	Protein (g)	Sugar (g)	Fiber (g)	Fat (g)	Sodium (mg)
Grilled Salmon with Yogurt Sauce	1 fillet	182	25	5.3	0.8	6.9	112
Catalan Fish	100 g	212	31	11	3.6	4.7	446

Pastas and Pizzas

Herb and Lemon Orzo	200 ml	240	7.8	45	1.9	2.8	4.5
Pan Fusilli	400 ml	305	21	40	7.2	9.2	381
Pizza Dough	1 slice	249	8.9	50	5.9	2.2	585
Pizza Party! (margharita)	1 wedge	336	17	52	6.1	7.4	816
Roast Pepper and Chicken Pasta	400 ml	454	19	49	2	20	302
Presto Tuna and Tomato Pasta	400 ml	368	24	49	1.4	7	336
Creamy Pesto Sauce Pasta	500 ml	521	20	68	4	17	276
Parmesan Polenta	150 ml	133	6.2	18	1.1	3.9	550
Deluxe Tomato Ravioli	300 ml	528	20	82	4.5	14	1141
Tortellini with Ratatouille Sauce	300 ml	358	13	57	3.5	9.1	394
Clam Linguine	500 ml	402	23	59	2	6.2	91

Vegetarian

Crispy Tofu	125 g	315	21	10	2.9	23	258

Recipes	Per Serving	Calories	Protein (g)	Sugar (g)	Fiber (g)	Fat (g)	Sodium (mg)
Mozzarella Carrozza	1 sandwich	378	21	40	3,7	16	690
East Indian Chick Peas	250 ml	250	10	43	5.6	5.3	36
Mushroom, Spinach and Feta Barley	250 ml	252	10	41	5	6.5	479

Eggs

Broccoli Frittata	1 wedge	182	15	6.8	0.9	10	580
Eggs à La Carte (Ham and Cheese)	1 toast	261	20	15	1.6	14	763
Potato Frittata	1 wedge	234	12	22	2.8	11	684
Greek Quiche	1 wedge	324	13	29	1.2	18	603

Desserts

Fresh Cheese Crêpes	1 crêpe	88	4.1	14	0.3	2	70
The Smoothy	250 ml	210	11	37	0.7	3.1	168
Decorator Cake Delight	1 square	243	3.9	43	1.2	7.9	121
Date and Orange Squares	1 square	282	3.3	46	3.2	10	65
Raspberry Cream	125 ml	61	2.9	8.6	1.1	1.7	3.5

Recipes	Per Serving	Calories	Protein (g)	Sugar (g)	Fiber (g)	Fat (g)	Sodium (mg)
Pear Yogurt Squares	1 square	350	6.9	51	1.6	14	120
Maple Pudding	125 ml	149	4.9	27	0.1	2.6	67

Fruit Variations

Vanilla Apples	1/2 apple	110	0.2	28	1.4	0.3	5.3
Homemade Jello	125 ml	58	1.9	13	0.9	0.2	3.5
Vanilla Apple Sauce	125 ml	180	0.5	45	4	0.8	4.5
Grilled Fruit	1 fruit	89	0.5	23	2.9	0.5	0.1
Tropical Sherbert	125 ml	47	1.8	9.6	1	0.6	23

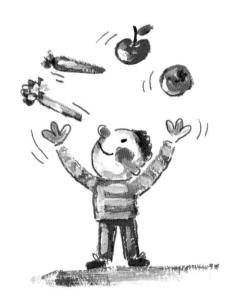

Index

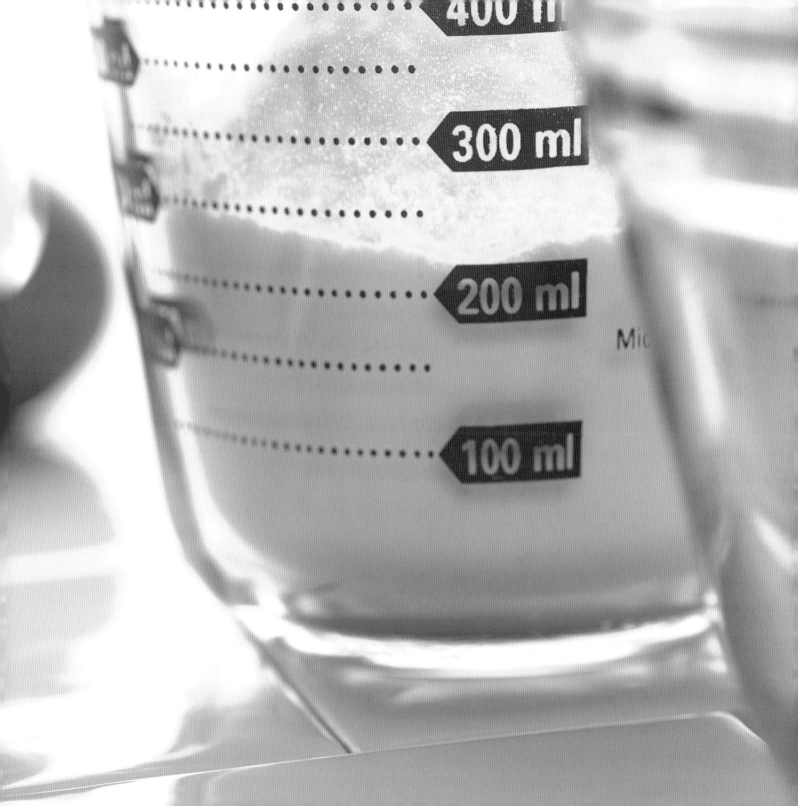